Miracle Lady on 6th Floor

One Woman's Survival Through
Cancer, Its Aftereffects
And Near-Death Experience

By

Ruth E. Foat

ISBN: 0-7596-9079-0

This book is printed on acid free paper.

1stBooks - rev. 01/10/02

Dedication

I lovingly dedicate this book to my Hero, Jesus Christ, who bore the stripes for my healing and to all those who prayed for me during the various stages of physical attacks on my body. You intercessors did not give up! You are among my most treasured gifts from God.

Contents

Acknowledgements

- I am indebted to my husband, Arvy, who not only prayed for me, but lovingly and without complaint completely cared for me, plus doing all the cooking, cleaning, shopping, and laundry.

- To my children and their families (Mary, Nancy, Sheryl, and Roger) for their constant reassurance, love, concern, and prayers. They continually requested prayer at their home churches and notified other friends.

- To my extended family, friends, and Pastor Close for their prayers, confidence in God, phone calls, cards, encouragement, and financial help.

- To Helen Rule for her insight and assistance. She exemplifies a true believer.

- To the Cancer Treatment Centers of America/Tulsa Tumor Board for their persistence in choosing the right methods of treatment and their loving, supportive, wholesome care.

- To Dr. David Wakefield, Ph.D. and Dr. Gerald Ellingson, Ph.D, Psychologists, for their prayers, insights, probing questions, and loving guidance.

- To Dr. Richard Sidwell, surgeon, for tackling an impossible situation. And to the Mercy Medical Center critical care team for their profound efforts to save my life.

- To Stanley and Lois Hankins for giving of their time and expertise in correcting my grammar.

Forward

Our church is filled with trophies. They are not baseball, basketball, or contest trophies. They are trophies of God's grace. Because we all must ask the question, "Where would I be if it wasn't for Jesus?" When we truly contemplate the implications of that question we recognize how dependent upon Christ we really are.

Ruth Foat is one of our more marvelous trophies. She is a trophy of God's miraculous power and His healing ability. It has been a privilege to pray for Ruth and believe with her during part of the events recorded in the chapters of this book. We prayed for her as she left for Tulsa and while she was there. We prayed for her as she returned. I was there in the waiting room, in Mason City, when the doctor told us of the severity of the situation. I saw the concern on his face as he tried to draw a mental picture of exactly what was going on. I was there when he returned.

I am reminded of the answer a man gave to a questioning group of skeptics many years ago. He said, "One thing I do know. I was blind but now I see!" So often we desire the miraculous intervention of God before we even know whether or not we are actually going blind. We are headed in for tests and call the church to pray for a good report. I believe God often immediately answers these cries to Him. The only problem is it is easy for skeptics to doubt. They say, "You never were going blind in the first place." Ruth's story is not that kind of story. God's hand is visible. Ruth is an example of God working His miraculous power to heal and to take through the very shadow of death. These two are not opposed to each other. Neither of these two are statements of a lack of faith. God heals and God takes us through.

I know that your faith will be increased as you read this tale of a trophy. I pray that God will use these words to help you trust in Him no matter what you may be going through. God has helped Ruth and God will help you!

Clifford O. Close, Pastor
First Assembly of God
Mason City, Iowa

Prologue

My granddaughter, Jessica, asked some "probing" questions while I was writing this book.

"Grandma, why did God chose to heal you and why are others not healed?"

"Grandma, a group of kids I meet with every week are studying the book of James. What are your thoughts about James 5:14-15?"

"Is anyone among you sick? Let him call for the elders of the church, and let them pray over him, anointing him with oil in the name of the Lord. And the prayer of faith will save the sick, and the Lord will raise him up."

Since this is a story and not a Bible study, it does not list in study form the keys to healing and various reasons why one may or may not be healed. However, if the book is read carefully, the reader will see many keys to healing. I try to share honestly the dealings, the misconceptions, and pruning process that came about during my physical struggle, plus share the hope and keys to survival. May everyone who reads this be inspired to move forward in his or her personal walk with Jesus Christ.

Introduction

What a revelation! The Lord is willing and waiting for us to come to Him for repeated and constant infillings of Himself. Our pursuit of the Lord is always successful because He is forever seeking to reveal Himself to us. It is for increasing degrees of Him that we pray, for a more perfect awareness of the divine Presence. God's presence is everywhere. Jacob was not aware of the Lord's presence until he saw a vision of God and declared, "*Surely the Lord is in this place and I knew it not*" (Genesis 28:16).

When Charles Finney saw the decline in revival in 1845, he noted that converts were not so deeply humbled and quickened and thoroughly baptized with the Holy Spirit and continual infillings. He related that just as one meal does not satisfy human physical needs forever, so one baptism of the Holy Spirit is not sufficient for the spiritual necessities of life. He felt through deeper and deeper baptisms of the Holy Spirit, people are able to more completely embrace Christ in all His fullness. These fresh baptisms do not make people prefect, rather they enable people to progressively make greater attainments and be changed from "*glory to glory.*" (II Corinthians 3:18)

On the day of Pentecost (Acts 2) the disciples prayed in one accord and received the Baptism of the Holy Spirit. However, two chapters later, Peter senses their need for fresh infilling and leads a prayer meeting where he utters this mighty prayer:

> "*Now, Lord, look on their threats, and grant to Your servants that with all boldness they may speak Your word, by stretching out Your hand to heal, and that signs and wonders may be done through the name of Your*

holy Servant Jesus. And when they had prayed, the place where they were assembled together was shaken; and they were all filled with the Holy Spirit, and they spoke the word of God with boldness" (Acts 4:29-31).

Has the church been conditioned to believe that the work of God will grow and souls will be won by finding the latest technique or secret? Only additional empowerment will help the church deal with this threat. After Pentecost, Peter preached and thousands came to Christ. Yet two chapters later he is drawing the church together for a fresh infilling. Peter rightly declared that the threat was from Satan. The church is under supernatural siege and only supernatural power can deliver it. Peter did not pray for personal safety, for emotional blessing, or for protection from hurt, gossip, or malicious alignment, but for boldness to preach. His passion was for the Word of God to have full impact on the lost and hurting.

For the church at Ephesus, Paul prays,
  "May He grant you out of the rich treasure of His glory to be strengthened and reinforced with mighty power in the inner man by the (Holy) Spirit [Himself]— indwelling your innermost being and personality... That you may be filled (through all your being) unto all the fullness of God—[that is] may you have the richest measure of the divine Presence, and become a body wholly filled and flooded with God Himself (Ephesians 3:16,19b Amplified)!

Again, Paul exhorts the Colossians to
  "Have the roots [of your being] firmly and deeply planted [in Him]—fixed and founded in Him—being continually built up in Him, becoming increasingly more confirmed and established in the faith, just as you were taught, and abounding and overflowing in it with thanksgiving" (Colossians 2:7 Amplified).

Throughout Paul's writings one is able to discern his heart cry for the churches to continually be built up in the Lord, to be entirely filled and flooded with God Himself, and to be strengthened with mighty power by the Holy Spirit's indwelling presence.

Like Moses' crying, "*Show me Your glory*" (Exodus 33:18), like Paul's writing, "*That I may know Him and the power of His resurrection…*" (Philippians 3:10), and like Peter's admonition "*to grow in the grace and knowledge of our Lord and Savior Jesus Christ*" (II Peter 3:18) has been the yearning of my heart for several years. I want to be filled with His divine Presence daily and walk in His continual fresh anointing.

A quote from some speaker written in the front of my Bible says, "We never change unless we are miserable." Never could I have imagined what lie ahead to cause many changes to take place in my life.

Mother's Caregiver

Chapter 1

The summer of 1997 marked the beginning of events that would profoundly change my life. The first week of September, my Mother called asking if I could come and help. Her husband was in the hospital. He could not come home without someone being there to help take care of him. Neither my mother nor my stepfather were able to care for themselves any longer. He passed away within a short time, and Mother came to live with me. About six months before this episode, I told Arvy, my husband, that I felt the Lord was showing me that I would be caring for her. I had prayed and made a commitment that I would honor her, and sweetly and lovingly take care of her before she even came to my home.

Mother was so happy living with us. She dreaded and feared going to a nursing home. She loved being with her family. The winter was much milder in southern Missouri than where she lived in Iowa. This made it possible for her to get out more. I would bundle her up with a heavy coat, scarf, and gloves so that we could take a little walk on most days. She loved to sit in a chair outside on warm fall days and watch me clean out the flowerbeds and trim back the bushes. In the spring, she would sit on the back deck and watch me work in the garden.

Our dining room had glass patio doors going out onto a deck. Because Mother loved watching birds Arvy made a form out of pipe and hooked it onto the deck railing. On that we hung several bird feeders with various types of food and suet. Mother would sit for hours at a time watching the birds, and she enjoyed identifying the ones she didn't know from a bird book. One summer day Mother got very excited while watching a cardinal bring its young to the feeders. The cardinal would break open the sunflower seed and pop it into the baby's mouth as the baby continued to fuss the whole time it was preparing another seed. The downy woodpeckers especially liked the suet, along with the red-breasted woodpecker; occasionally a pilated woodpecker would stop by. We identified over 30 bird species that first winter. Cardinals were Mother's favorite because of their beauty. Often there were eight to ten on the deck at the same time.

Saturday morning was bath time for Mother, which she dreaded, because she would get so cold. I would turn the thermostat up plus run an electric heater for an hour before starting her bath. Arvy had taken the tub/shower out and put in a large shower with just a short lip to step across to make it easier for her to get in and out. After getting her into the shower onto a bath stool, I would run the water as warm as she could stand and quickly shampoo and bathe her. The sweat would drip off of me as I worked in that hot steamy room. She was always glad when the shower was done and warm clothes were on. Her Saturday ritual, following her shower, was to choose one of her favorite videos to watch, which frequently was Anne of Green Gables.

We stayed home the first Christmas Mother was with us because she did not want to go north in the cold weather. Even though we kept the thermostat up, she wore long underwear and sweat suits plus having a throw over her a lot of the time to keep warm.

The next summer I took her north to my brother's farm, and they planned a big 86th birthday party for her. Then her other two daughters took her for a few weeks, which allowed her to visit most of her grandchildren as well as all of her children that summer. Looking back, we are very glad she did because it was her last summer with us.

That fall at Thanksgiving, both Mother's daughters and some of the grandchildren came to spend time with her. She enjoyed them so much. Mother continued to be happy, but I could see she was failing. She had fallen twice trying to get from the commode back into bed; consequently, a baby monitor was put into her room so that she could call me at night. Frequently, I had to get up and help her onto the commode and help her back into bed as she could no longer get out of bed alone or go to the bathroom alone.

Gradually her care required more and more time as she grew weaker. I knew the Lord put me into this situation. I had no idea how confining it would become, nor how many years this would go on. Mother got very sensitive about my being gone; she wanted someone with her all the time, even if she was napping. The last four months I was away from home only one hour on Sunday to teach Children's Church and an hour to purchase groceries each week. Arvy would teach an adult Sunday School class and return home to be with Mother while I led Children's Church. I was committed to take care of Mother for however long she lived, but I was questioning my strength to continue. I wore a lift belt so I could hold more weight and learned techniques to make sure she wouldn't fall getting out of the shower. She also lost her desire to take walks outside, as it was getting more difficult for her.

But a strange stirring was taking place in my spirit. During the fall of 1998, the Lord stirred my heart in several areas of study. Also I was fascinated in developing a series of notes on wilderness experiences. None of this made any sense because of my commitment to care for Mother.

Prophecies and prayers were spoken over me that seemed to confirm there was ministry in the future. I remembered crying out to the Lord, "I don't want to be set on a shelf or be content with retirement; I want to be in Your ministry. Are You using this time to build character in me?"

In my journal there were several expressions like: "I am so hungry for more of Jesus." Consequently, when a sermon was given regarding moving beyond complacency to compassionate renewal and new beginnings, it piqued my interest. The essence of the message declared the Lord is doing a new pruning of the branches, a new refining of the silver, a new blowing out the chaff, and a new circumcision of the heart. To have new beginnings, the Lord wants to refine us as silver; in other words, we go through the fire to surface imbedded areas that need to be cleaned out. The Lord also wants to blow out the chaff, which may be our defense mechanisms or offenses, and to circumcise our hearts from the fleshly ways of thinking or living. My response was, "Okay, Lord, I'm ready".

In our garden was a particular type of raspberry bush that had to be cut off every year at ground level and destroyed to make room for new growth. As I was cutting my raspberry canes and burning them, suddenly the Lord said to me, "I'm cutting away the old even though it produced fruit so that it will produce more fruit." Pruning in my mind was for branches that were getting old or were not producing. Suddenly I remembered before cutting off the raspberry canes, I had picked about a quart of berries. The summer after cutting them to the ground, there was an abundant crop. We ate raspberries at nearly every meal for two months and had eight gallons in the freezer.

As I pondered what the Lord shared with me in the raspberry garden, I wondered what it meant. The Lord seemed to be saying that He was going to cut everything away. I asked the Lord, "What do You intend to do with me?" I felt that everything the Lord had ever spoken to me was being pruned. This had such a profound effect on me that I kept a bonfire going several days burning notes and Bible studies that I had developed over the years. I wanted to be ready for something new. If the Lord ever wanted to use me again in teaching or speaking, apparently He would give me a fresh word.

Then I read John 15:2 in the Amplified: "*Any branch in Me that does not bear fruit—that stops bearing—He cuts away (trims off, takes away). And He cleanses and repeatedly prunes every branch that continues to bear fruit, to make it bear more and richer and more excellent fruit.*" It became clear that all the fruit or influence or good that had happened through my life was being cut off at ground level, in order that He could do a new thing. "*And the remnant ... shall again take root downward, and bear fruit upward*" (Isaiah 37:31). "*Enlarge the place of your tent, and let them stretch out the curtains of your habitations; do not spare; lengthen your cords, and strengthen your stakes*" (Isaiah 54:2).

I wondered what the Lord had in mind? We were on an exciting journey together.

Emergency Message

Chapter 2

At the beginning of December 1998, I was scheduled for an annual physical exam. The night before the appointment I started hemorrhaging. The doctor said that everything looked fine, but he did proceed with the pap test. I was uneasy because the hemorrhaging continued all through December. Also, it was getting more difficult physically to care for Mother. I wasn't sure if it was because Mother was weaker, or if it was because I was weaker. The truth was that both of us were getting weaker.

I had been taking care of Mother for nearly a year and a half and had missed last Christmas with the family, due to her living with us. My sister graciously offered to care for her during the week of Christmas this year, so we could be with our family. December flew by with the usual rush of Christmas season, caring for Mother, and packing her things, and getting her ready to go. After taking Mother to my sister's home in Illinois, we went to Iowa to spend Christmas with our children and grandchildren. It was a special joyous occasion, since we had missed being with them last year.

When we arrived home, an emergency message was on the answering machine asking me to call immediately. The nurse told me the pap was bad and showed cancer. When I questioned her further, she admitted it was a stage four cancer—very serious. I was scheduled to go to another city to see a specialist and have further tests the first week of January.

My sister brought Mother back to our home before New Year's because a storm was forecast. We discussed my medical situation, and she agreed that she would arrange for help to take care of Mother for a while, if necessary. She is a teacher and knew she couldn't leave Mother alone all day.

While riding a bicycle in New Orleans, our son was hit by a truck. At the same time, my youngest daughter was in the middle of divorce. She is a mother of four teenagers, ages 15, 14, and 13 year old twins. I was very grieved for her and the grandchildren. I wondered how she could survive all the new responsibilities? How could she support them? She married very young and worked while her husband got his degree, which left her without higher education.

The news about our son's accident, the news about our daughter's divorce, and the news of cancer all within a few days of each other were overwhelming. Faith in a living God was my ultimate source of strength. Faith is not a bridge over troubled waters, but a pathway through them. *"Many are the afflictions of the righteous, but the Lord delivers him out of them all"* (Psalms 34:19). The Lord didn't promise deliverance from trials, but He assured deliverance through them. When the Lord says "not now" or "not yet" that does not mean no. I knew that Jesus Christ was my Lord. Who else could possibly do what He can do? Who else could see me through this situation? In Philippians Paul says, *"so now also Christ will be magnified in my body, whether by life or by death. For to me, to live is Christ, and to die is gain"* (Philippians 1:20c-21). For me, this is a win win situation. I trusted Him completely.

Tests were done throughout the month of January. During the month Psalms 23 became daily restoration for my soul. My brother-in-law, a messianic Jew, sent me a literal translation from the Hebrew of Psalm 23. It blessed me greatly; here it is:

7

Because Yahwey the Lord, our healer, our provider,
our peace, or righteous shepherd,
our indwelling presence, our banner,
is our shepherd,
I shall never be squeezed for anything.
He will lay me down among the living pastures.
By the living peaceful waters he pushes and guides me.
He gives me back my soul, my spirit and my life.
*H*e takes me, and places me in the straight paths of truth
And righteousness because of His names sake,
Who is Jesus Christ.
Even though I go through the veil of death,
I have no fear of anything evil happening to me,
Because You are standing with me and upholding me,
Your rod and staff bring me your mercy.
You have prepared a table for me
In the presence of my adversaries,
You have anointed my head with so much of your oil
It runs all over me.
I know for a fact that Your goodness,
And Your love, and Your mercy will chase me
All the days of my life
And I will sabbath in the house of the Lord
All the days of my life.

Two months of hemorrhaging had taken a toll. My sister-in-law told me she thought I was going to die before the doctors decided upon a procedure. *"Therefore we do not become discouraged—utterly spiritless, exhausted, and wearied out through fear. Though our outer man is (progressively) decaying and wasting away, yet our inner self is being (progressively) renewed day after day"* (II Corinthians 4:16 Amplified). This verse and the Lord is my Shepherd was a lifeline of reassurance. Two nights before the diagnosis was determined, the Lord gave me an indescribable peace.

Mother was quite distraught when I had to go to the hospital for a dilatation and curettage (D&C) procedure. My sister-in-law stayed with her all day, and they watched some of Mother's favorite videos. When I awoke following the D&C procedure on January 27, 1999, the doctor told me that the lining of my uterus was full of cancer. He scheduled a total hysterectomy for the following week. Immediately, arrangements had to be made for Mother's care plus all the packing of her clothes, medication, and medical equipment, which had to be taken to my sister. When I kissed Mother goodbye, I assured her I would try to get her home in six weeks' time.

The day following the hysterectomy, CT scans and x-rays were taken of an area by the aorta that the doctors were concerned about. The oncology radiologist scrubbed in for the surgery to check the area and, he seemed pleased that the tests turned out normal. They told me there would be five weeks of radiation following the recovery time.

I was home four days when violent vomiting began. By the next day, I could hardly get out of bed. I was so sick. During that time a card came with life-giving thoughts: "To let you know that there are many of us praying for you! We are standing with you, fighting for you! Our God Reigns! He is Lord of all! Our confidence is in Him! He is faithful! I speak Life to you in Jesus' name!" Those words brought so much life to me. Tears poured down my face as the Lord ministered to my heart.

The following morning my husband called the doctor, and Arvy was instructed to take me to the emergency room immediately, an hour's drive away. After seven hours in the emergency room during which my stomach was being pumped, tests were being taken, and doctors were contemplating another surgery; the decision was finally made that there was a bowel blockage. They put me in the hospital for three more days while the stomach pump continued. Finally, the bowels began to function. During the emergency room time, the nurse kept commenting about the peace I had. It wasn't me. I was so sick that all I could say was, "Lord, You are my shepherd." There had to be intercessors praying, as I was too weak to pray.

Within a week of returning home from the hospital, a call came that Mother was put into the hospital with pneumonia. She was in such a weakened condition; her family was greatly concerned that she would not recover.

Enemy Came In Like A Flood

Chapter 3

Within couple of weeks of Mother's initial hospitalization, the family realized she would not survive. Despite the fact that I was not strong following surgery, we made the five-hour trip to visit her at the hospital. Even though she was in a coma, the family stood around her bed and sang hymns to her. It was obvious she was touched as we watched her facial muscles visibly relax. A week before she went into a deep coma, she shared several things she was witnessing. She saw heaven and said, "It's so wonderful, I can't believe it."

I went to the drug store to return some of Mother's unopened prescriptions; however, they could not take them back. As I stood there, the overwhelming emotion of her condition and near departure hit me. Tears rolled down my cheeks, which surprised me, as I'm not inclined to do that in a public place. Then I walked past the isle where I purchased her Depends and other supplies; again tears flowed. Later when I took a shower, tears ran as I remembered all the special care for her in that place. I wasn't very strong physically and tears came easily.

On March 22, five weeks after surgery for uterine cancer, we had to go to a major cancer center, to see the radiology oncology doctor. He discussed the seriousness of the cancer. It was much worse than I had previously been told. He explained the side effects of radiation and wanted to start the radiation immediately. As tears welled in my eyes, I told him my mother was in hospice and dying, and I asked if I could wait until the funeral was over. He agreed to wait but stated emphatically, "You need to see our

11

grief counselor because you are facing radiation, the death of your mother, and a funeral." Emotionally, I was about to fall apart, but I did not accept his proposal of visiting a counselor. I just wanted to get home to rest. He gave me literature to read and for the most part it discussed discouragement, despair, and hopelessness that arise during treatment.

I read the materials during the hour-long drive; and when we arrived home, I felt completely engulfed in an ominous black cloud. I was trained from youth on to practice self-discipline and struggled to be cheerful which is my natural disposition. But my mind and emotions were beyond any previous experience. No amount of prayer or personal resolve could block out the intense blackness and sense of helplessness I felt. Questions raged in my mind, "Would anything be normal again? How long would Mother suffer? Does death have to be like this? How will radiation affect me? Will I live through this?" Even in my anguish, I felt there had to be a way out. If a counselor could help me, surely God could see me through! *"...When the enemy comes in like a flood, the Spirit of the Lord will lift up a standard against him"* (Isaiah 59:19c).

Ironically, in the midst of the darkness and despair, the deep-settled peace of the Lord remained. What a paradox! Grief, two surgeries, a bowel blockage, and mother's dying process all within five weeks' time chipped away at my physical stamina. A false opinion in my thinking was if I read scriptures and maintained a prayer life, the enemy could not attack with such overwhelming sinister foreboding. But the combination of grief, surgery, and weakness had taken a great toll physically and emotionally.

A few days before this experience, two tapes on healing came in the mail from a friend. When they arrived, I hesitated to listen to them. Mentally, I couldn't handle a preacher telling me what to do or say; I was just too exhausted and weak. However, due to my dilemma, I changed my mind and listened to the tape and realized the speaker was reading the Word on healing—not preaching. As I listened to the healing scriptures and followed them in my Bible, life was ministered to me. Two verses especially became living rhema (fresh word) from the Lord to my heart: "*I shall not die, but live to declare the works of the Lord*" (Psalms 118:17). I knew that was a promise from the Lord, and the second verse dealt with my grief: "*He heals the broken-hearted and binds up their wounds*" (Psalms 147:3). The blackness lifted, but I was in for the fight of my life. Too many times we stop here and claim the promises, but we do not continue to "*fight the good fight of faith*" (I Timothy 6:12).

From that point on, I listened to or read or sang verses from the Bible several hours daily. Mother passed away four days later, and I listened to scripture tapes all the way to the funeral (600 miles) and back. Mother's funeral was a glorious home going. Several of her granddaughters sang. The husband of one granddaughter preached a message challenging all of the family to continue in the great spiritual heritage we had received. It was a blessed time together, even though we all missed her terribly. Now my responsibility shifted from caregiver and power of attorney to administrator of her will, and even the simplest tasks seemed overwhelming.

Immediately upon our return from the funeral, radiation treatments began. Healing Scriptures were played daily during the two-hour trip for radiation. I searched the Bible for more verses on "quicken" because in the Hebrew it means to live, to revive, to make alive, to give promise of life, and to restore to life. Psalms 119 has many verses declaring the effectiveness of the word; however, many also have provisions. "*I am afflicted very much; revive me, O Lord, according to Your word*" (Psalms 119:107). "*Let your heart retain my words, keep my commands, and live*" (Proverbs 4:4). Notice the conditions in the following Scripture:

"*My son,*
    (1) Give attention to my words,
    (2) Incline your ear to my sayings,

(3) Do not let them depart from your eyes,
(4) Keep them in the midst of your heart,

For they are life to those who find them and [radiant] health to all their flesh." (Proverbs 4:20-22) See Exodus 15:26 also.

The word of God always encouraged and caused me to feel better, even though the enemy challenged every step of faith achieved. The scripture tapes and reading of the Word were tremendous sources of strength through the weakening process of radiation.

I went forward in church for anointing and prayer before starting radiation. The pastor only prayed, "Be whole according to your faith." I went back to my seat and cried, "God you set me up, that's not what I wanted to hear." Questions flooded in like: "Will I have enough faith? What if I don't believe good enough?" The pastor's words really hit an area of struggle in my life.

Pruning was continuing to take place. The Lord wanted to clean out some misconceptions I had of myself. I wanted the pastor to pray in great faith and believe for my healing, because I mistrusted my ability to believe. The enemy was having a hay-day with my mind.

While Jesus was instructing the disciples about faith, He taught them to say to the mountain, "*Be removed and cast into the sea, and does not doubt in his heart, and believes that those things he says will come to pass, he will have whatever he says. Therefore I say to you, whatever things you ask when you pray, believe that you receive them, and you will have them*" (Mark 11:23-24).

The Lord began to show me that in my heart I had great confidence in the Him. The temptation to waver was in my mind: "Am I doing everything right?" There was absolutely no one else to put confidence in, to trust in, or to believe for healing, but our blessed Lord. I had to choose to rest in that and not beat myself up over my inadequacies.

A great little book for anyone with cancer, <u>Healed of Cancer</u> by Dodie Osteen, arrived shortly after I worked through the frustration over the word "doubt." Amazingly, this great lady of faith went through the same things about wavering. I could identify with the struggles she shared. She comments about feeling great condemnation when she wavered regarding the Lord healing her, even though it is a common element of a long struggle with sickness. Her husband asked her if she was wavering in her heart, and she said "no." What a confirmation of the same thing the Lord had shown me. It is easy to feel you are the only one who strives with such issues or that you are not saying or doing something right. Perhaps the enemy of our soul wants us to suppose others are strong, while we feel weak, debilitated, and exhausted.

The scriptures became my living source, and I spent many hours in the Word each day. *"But his delight is in the law of the Lord, and in His law (word) he meditates day and night. He shall be like a tree planted by the rivers of water, that brings forth its fruit in its season, whose leaf also shall not wither…"* (Psalm 1:2-3). In Hebrew thought, to meditate upon the scriptures is to quietly repeat them in a soft, droning sound, while utterly abandoning outside distractions. It is reciting texts, praying intense prayers, and getting lost in communion with God. The scriptures were my sustenance, my hope, my stability, and my life.

The last portion of Psalm 1:3 *"leaf shall not wither"* gave me hope as I remembered the leaves mentioned in Revelation. In heaven, *"the leaves of the tree were for the healing of the nations"* (Revelation 22:2c). The issue was not whether I would live or die; that was in His hands, and He had given me a promise. The issue was could I make it through strong in Him. I am learning, and will continue to learn, not to condemn myself. A tremendous deepening confidence in the Lord arose. A new assurance was taking place. God will take care of me while I walk in obedience and trust Him. *"I will meditate on your*

majestic, glorious splendor and your wonderful miracles"
(Psalm 145:5 NLT).

Restoration by Grace

Chapter 4

During each radiation treatment, I meditated on Psalm 23, The Lord's Prayer, and other verses. It was especially comforting to picture Jesus laying me down among the green pastures, listening to the peaceful waters, and believing He was anointing my head with so much of His oil that it was running all over me plus His love and mercy were chasing me all the days of my life. I continued the same process with The Lord's Prayer.

The process of radiation causes the body to become weaker and weaker. It caused relentless diarrhea in me. It was so out of control, the doctor stopped radiation for a week and instructed me to take 12-16 Imodium pills a day. Even that didn't stop the diarrhea, but it slowed it. Radiation was completed in six weeks, after which I could barely walk due to weakness. I remember the last day of radiation; I wondered if I had enough strength to walk from the car into the building for treatment.

Following radiation, I tried to do little things to build strength. I planted a garden by working only one short row a day. I took very short walks daily, which caused me to gasp for air. My legs could hardly move.

Two months later, I drove 600 miles to visit daughter Sheryl, who was recently divorced. I wanted to do something to encourage her in the Lord, to see her hurts healed, and to see her radiant again. I took her to a woman's conference in Fargo, and my sister and her daughter stayed in the same room with us. The younger ladies had wonderful fellowship, and Sheryl was ministered to mightily.

On the way home from the conference, we picked up Sheryl's twin boys, Matt and Luke. They were on their way home from church camp. I questioned them about camp until I knew that they had accepted Jesus. They told me that a camp counselor helped them understand what they had done in praying the sinner's prayer after watching a video that I had sent them. My heart was full of joy.

Since I was in Minnesota with Sheryl, Women's Aglow in Albert Lea asked me to share my experiences concerning my surgery and radiation. It was a blessed time, as I saw many long-time friends. The Lord moved in a special way. My heart was full to overflowing with gratitude for all the Lord had brought me through, for His anointing during ministry, and for time spent with dear friends.

About two weeks later, excruciating pain developed in the bursa in both hips from inflammation caused by the radiation. The doctor suggested taking twelve ibuprofen pills daily. Not wanting to tear up my stomach, I only took two at bedtime. I wondered how long I could withstand the torment. I couldn't bear to sit in church, didn't sleep well, and life was a miserable mountain of pain. I questioned the Lord, "Will I ever be free of pain?" When we pray for healing or deliverance through trials, the answer may not be instantaneous. The greatest relief of pain would come when I sat at the piano with an open Bible and sang the Psalms to the Lord, making up a melody. Singing along with Scripture music and reading the Scriptures helped, too.

Five months later, a lady invited me to a little home meeting. She informed me a pastor from another town was coming to speak about healing. I hesitated going due to pain. My husband eventually encouraged me to go. I took pillows to sit on and to put behind my back. The speaker spoke about healing using many of the verses I had memorized. The message stirred me deeply and faith burst forth in my heart. Three times during the message, he stopped, pointed toward me, and said, "This is your night; you are going to be healed." He had never heard of me, and I had never heard of him. Immediately after the message, he walked to me and prayed. From that moment on, the unbearable pain in the bursae left. To this day, the bursae remain inflamed and tender, but to a tolerable degree.

Jesus will speak to the mountain in our lives by His Spirit of Grace. "…*This [addition of the bowl to the candlestick, causing it to yield a ceaseless supply of oil from the olive trees] is the word of the Lord to Zerubbabel, saying, 'Not by might, nor by power, but by My Spirit [of Whom the oil is a symbol]', says the Lord of hosts. 'For who are you, O great mountain [of human obstacles]'"* (Zechariah 4:6-7a Amplified)? I am so glad for the Spirit of the Lord that deals with our obstacles and gives us a ceaseless supply of oil (His Spirit).

The enemy will do anything to keep us from moving forward. He will point out every imaginable mountain or invent mountains. As we go through pressures of life—disasters, crises, sicknesses, discouragement, etc.—we have a choice to become better or get bitter. The old adage states the same sun that melts butter hardens clay. "*So be truly glad! There is wonderful joy ahead even though it is necessary for you to endure many trials for a while. These trials are only to test your faith, to show that it is strong and pure. It is being tested as fire tests and purifies gold—and your faith is far more precious to God than mere gold. So if your faith remains strong after being tried by fiery trials, it will bring you much praise and glory and honor on the day when Jesus Christ is revealed to the whole world*" (I Peter 1:6-7 NLT).

Pressure and resistance builds muscle. My grandson lifts weights to strengthen his shoulders and arms for football. After many months he has bulging muscles. The Lord allows resistance to come against us to help us become strong that we may be able to stand. (Ephesians 6:11) Paul returned to cities he ministered in "*Establishing and strengthening the souls and the hearts of the disciples, urging and warning and encouraging them to stand firm in the faith, and telling them that it is through many hardships and tribulations we must enter the kingdom of*

God" (Acts 14:22 Amplified). The person with no trials has no triumphs.

Everyone wants to hear about the immunity that the blood of Jesus supplies, but many do not want to hear what it takes to walk in it. Let God strip us so that He can equip us. God wants to turn disaster into victory and barrenness into fruitfulness. Discouragements, disappointments, and distractions can cause us to forget the Lord's vision and dreams for us. But in each of our spiritual wombs is a seed of destiny waiting to be born.

Grace is not just a beginning, but also a lifelong way to live. I read a story about a godless village. When someone does something wrong, the villagers gather in a large circle and put the offender in the middle of the circle. Each one around the circle steps up one at a time and points a finger at the offender and reminds him of a thing he has done right. What a picture of restoration by grace. I believe people want most to hear, "I love you," "I forgive you," and "come have a cup of coffee with me." Isn't that a picture of our precious Savior? "I love you, I forgive you, come and dine," Jesus says.

"*And some of those who are wise, prudent and understanding shall be weakened and fall; [thus then the insincere among the people will lose courage and become deserters. It will be a test] to refine, to purify and makes those among [God's people] white, even to the time of the end; because it is yet for the time God appointed*" (Daniel 11:35 Amplified). Daniel is pointing out that even wise, sensible, and good people will fall; but the Lord will refine, purify, and restore them in the end. Oh, that we would walk in that kind of grace, encouraging and restoring one another, instead of pointing fingers of accusation.

Moving North?

Chapter 5

Our children suggested that we move closer to one of them. Each of our four children live in different states, but all felt our best choice would be to move near the two daughters, one in Iowa and one in Minnesota. Mary, a diabetic, particularly had prayed we would move nearer. She went so far as to inform us she felt it was the Lord's will that we move to Mason City. Why would God tell our daughter such a thing, or was it her imagination? Wouldn't He speak to us first (normal parental feelings-smile)?

That was unsettling for us because we didn't want to move. We enjoyed the warmer climate near Branson. The doctors who were treating me were in that area, and Arvy had a good part-time locksmith business. On the other hand, people in our community often moved closer to their children as they got older and needed their children's help.

Arvy had recently lost his brother to heart failure and older sister to brain cancer. His younger sister and only sibling left, lived a half mile from us. We were together a lot and it would be difficult for all of us to be many miles apart. We walked together frequently or had coffee with each other. Arvy always talked by phone with his sis Marlene every day.

Eventually, we listed our home with a realtor trying to find out if this was the Lord's will. After three months of no activity on the house, we took it off the market and thought, "This must not be God's direction." It was late fall and we did not want to move in winter. Nevertheless, at this time we were still

21

bewildered about what we should do, but we were willing to follow the Lord's leading. For that reason we prayed, "Lord, regarding this house and a move, we don't know your will. Please open the doors so wide that we know it is You, or close them so tight, we know that is You." We put it in His hands and the confusion left us. Wonderful peace settled over our thinking and emotions.

Approximately a month later a realtor from a different town called. He asked, "Is your house off the market?" Arvy's "yes" didn't dissuade him. He continued, "I have a couple sitting across the desk from me who want to live on your street. Would you let me show them your house because it seems to meet the qualifications they desire?"

Arvy agreed to let them look. They were not in the house ten minutes when I surmised they wanted to purchase it. They loved everything: the color of the carpets, the layout, the big kitchen, the deck, the double garage, the nice shed, and the size of the double lot. I had planted pear, cherry, nectarine, apricot, and peach trees, as well as blueberry and raspberry bushes, a raised strawberry bed, and a nice garden plot. Most places in the area had none of these amenities.

To our amazement, shortly after the people toured the house, the realtor came back with a contract. The purchasers wanted to occupy the home within six weeks, which would be mid-January. We laughed as it sank into our thinking; this must be the Lord's direction; and we would have to move in the winter. Here we were trying to get out of moving in the winter, and the Lord knew we would all along. What a joke on us! The Lord must have a sense of humor!

We went to Marlene's home to share our news. It was a sad time for her, even though it was obviously the Lord's timing for us to move. We had no idea why the Lord wanted us to move, but we desired to follow His leading.

Immediately, I started packing. I was still in a weakened condition and was unable to work more than couple of hours at a time and then rest. Arvy decided to drive his pickup and pull a

U Haul trailer to Iowa at Christmas time, instead of driving the car. He stored his wood-working equipment, tractor mower, and many tools, at my brother's farm, making moving day much easier.

Christmas seemed very rushed. It was a precious time with the children and grandchildren. Only our son was unable to be there. We were in Iowa about three days and hurried back home to continue packing. Arvy also was helping a locksmith friend with his business, which put even more pressure on our getting packed. The weather permitted us to have a yard sale, and we advertised some furniture in the paper. We were scaling down our things, so that we could live in a smaller home.

On moving day the truck was loaded by mid-afternoon with the help of some dear friends. Our plan was to leave the next morning, but due to a forecast of rain and icy roads developing that evening, we left immediately. In the Ozarks, ice is particularly treacherous. We drove enough hours to be north of the ice storm and dropped into a motel bed exhausted. We had to press on quickly the next morning because a blizzard was forecast for that evening in northern Iowa, our destination. Wasn't the Lord good? He helped us to get through between the storms.

We put everything into storage except for bedroom furniture, which we moved into a room at our son-in-law and daughter's home. This arrangement was a mutual benefit to both of us, as we had a place to live while looking for a home, and our living with them took some of the workload off Mary. At the time she had been a diabetic 38 years, and it had taken a toll on her physically. While living with them, the children did not have to go to daycare, and I helped them with their homework. Also I cooked the evening meal, cleaned the house, and did most of the laundry.

We contacted a realtor to locate a house for us. Our price range didn't leave much in quality homes. The houses we looked at were extremely old with steep stairways to the second floor, and not at all what we wanted. It would be impossible for us to make house payments on social security, and neither of us was physically able to work much. When the realtor asked how our home sold in Missouri, we shared the story of how we prayed.

In March, Mary was invited to a Thyme In The Kitchen home party. I went along and it was a lot of fun. The consultant made quite an impression on me, plus she was witty and personable. I wondered if this was something I could do at my own pace, without an investment, to help with the cost of prescriptions. She met me and explained the program and a way to earn my starter kit without cost. I wanted a few days to consider the proposal; consequently, she invited me to a class.

Helen took me to a cooking class in Minneapolis at the headquarters of Thyme In The Kitchen. I met several other consultants, and she introduced me to the president. Judy, the president asked, "What is your greatest need?"

Immediately, I answered, "We need a home in our price range." Every home we looked into was in miserable condition or had a steep stairway to the bedrooms upstairs.

She replied, "I will intercede for you."

That evening, I pulled up the local realtor page on the Internet, and a new listing caught my eye. The next day the morning paper had an ad of the same listing with an open house. We toured it and liked what we saw. When the realtor came with a contract, she commented, "This must be the Lord." Previously, she had asked how we had sold our house and was aware that we had prayed. Then she stated that she had looked for something like this for two years for a friend and had not located anything. She had not seen the listing and was amazed we had found it. Again we felt the Lord had provided: this time, a small two bedroom older home on one floor.

The summer was extremely busy. I planned a family reunion on the Fourth of July, provided daycare for two of my grandchildren, and began developing my business with Thyme In the Kitchen. The family reunion was to be at my brother's farm, and he and his wife carried the bulk of the work. I did as much as I could, but I was not feeling well. We were surprised to see two cousins that we hadn't seen for over 40 years. All our immediate family came and many of the grandchildren. My brother and wife had made great effort for the grandchildren to have fun and had set up all kinds of games and things for the children to do in their spacious yard.

Near the end of July, I attended the Thyme In The Kitchen (TITK) annual convention. It was such an inspiring and fun time. Frequently a bell would ring, and gifts were given to all of us, as well as special drawings for gifts. We were treated like queens, and they provided us with great dining. The finale was a banquet and many awards were given. For the previous month, I won two second place awards after being in the business only three months. How exciting!

In August, TITK planned a special promotion month for the consultants and hostesses. They had produced new catalogs with new products for us, and I was on my way. It turned out to be my greatest month with over $5,000 in sales. That promoted me into a better position with the company. I was excited about building a business at my own pace that would help us financially.

However, I still suffered pain across the abdomen frequently and surmised it was from the radiation. A lot of the time I didn't feel well and had to push myself to keep up with all the bookings. However, the last week of August I realized the pain was worse, and I was getting weaker. Helen, my manager, realized it too, and she offered to drive and help me with my last demo of the month. I was barely able to stand long enough for an hour demo and had to quickly sit to rest awhile.

In the meantime, Arvy had been suffering with diarrhea and vomiting all summer; and after several visits to Mayo Clinic, they discovered he was reacting to some medication. Also, they found his potassium level to be dangerously high, and he was near kidney failure; actually he was very near death. The doctors were in the process of getting him on insulin and taking care of the other problems near the end of August. My concern was so great for him that I had not stopped to analyze my physical condition.

Oh! No! Not Again!

Chapter 6

My good friend, Helen, was preparing to go to the Cancer Treatment Centers of American/Tulsa for her six-month checkup. She had spoken highly of the center on several occasions and asked if I would like to go along. I decided to go, even though my oncologist in Missouri said I could wait a year before another check up; and this would be three months early. We left Iowa on Labor Day, September 4, 2000.

The cancer center is amazing. They treat the whole person through a combination of medical, nutritional, physical, psychological and spiritual therapies. They do so in a compassionate, caring environment that encourages patients to actively participate in important decisions about the management of their disease. The first two days were filled with blood tests, bone scans, CT scans, and doctor appointments. The oncologist was shocked that I had been told to wait a year before getting a check up. Also, I visited with the homeopathy doctor, and he explained the blood test results, which showed extremely low protein levels and anemia. I assumed that was the reason for recent weakness and he recommended things to build both to better levels.

September 8 was the appointment with the oncologist to learn the results of all the tests. Helen asked if I would like her to come along. I was so naïve that it never dawned on me that there could be a reason the protein and iron levels were so low. Helen, a former nurse, was suspicious; thank God she was with me. Dr. Nevinny reported a large mass of 5 ½" by 7 ½" in my abdomen. It was wrapped around the small intestine, the main vein went through it, and it was very close to the aorta. What a shock! No wonder I had been in pain, and it had continually been getting worse during the last two months.

Since the first cancer was in the uterus, I was sent across town to a gynecologist for an exam. He recommended a needle biopsy and surgery immediately. His prognosis was very shocking, and it was hard for me to comprehend the situation. Helen helped me sort through my uneasiness; I was very thankful she was along! When we arrived back at the cancer center, I requested a second opinion from their head surgeon. Since it was late Friday afternoon, they scheduled it for Monday. On the way back to the room, we met Jim, Helen's husband, coming off the elevator. I fell into his arms and cried.

When I called Arvy that evening to give him the report, he was not surprised. While he was driving home after delivering some grandchildren to camp, the Lord had dropped a word into his heart that I was getting a bad report. He had more appointments scheduled at Mayo and came to Tulsa as soon as those were finished.

Jim does outreach ministry for Wycliff Translators and had meetings scheduled during the weekend; therefore, Helen went with him. They asked me to go along, but I needed time to rest, time to listen to Scripture tapes, and time to pray. On Sunday, I visited Victory Christian Center. Their pastor had been in our home twenty years before and ministered at the church we pastored. He prayed for me, gave me a book on healing, and a tape of healing scripture songs. On the visitor's card I mentioned I was staying at the cancer center. A week later the church began sending volunteers to my room to pray and that continued throughout my stay.

After the surgeon examined me, he insisted on more tests. The mass was so big and in a dangerous location; consequently, he was very skeptical of doing a needle biopsy. He felt a biopsy would be extremely dangerous, and I might bleed to death. Whew! I was extremely grateful Helen had encouraged me to ask for a second opinion. During the next two weeks, there were upper GI tests, more CT Scans, and two MRI tests. A doctor and nutritionist brought sample protein drinks to my room and educated me to drink them three times a day to restore nutrients that the cancer had been sapping from my body. In the meantime, I was attending healing classes held at the Cancer Center by Rhema Bible School, attending Victory Christian Center every time possible, attending humor groups, and going to imaging classes conducted by a Christian psychologist.

In the beginning I hesitated going to an imaging class, wondering if it was scripturally correct. Some believers have shied away from meditation because Satan has used it in other forms. He does not create or invent anything new, but perverts that which God has already designed. What a clever ploy the enemy uses to either scare Christians from a good thing or to ensnare them with his trap.

Upon the death of Moses the Lord spoke specific encouragement and direction to Joshua in verses 1:2-9. How would you like to follow the greatest leader Israel ever had? The Lord knew Joshua's dilemma and emphasized the importance of meditation: "*The Book of the Law shall not depart from your mouth, but you shall meditate in it day and night…*" (Joshua 1:7) Psalm 1:2 also instructs us to meditate on His Word day and night.

The same can be said for imaging. Satan cunningly uses images of violence or a ten second sex scene to lure people into sin. The old saying "a picture speaks more than 10,000 words" is so true. Pornography on the Internet or videos, in magazines, and on TV is enticing thousands into perversion.

Jesus is the master imager. He spoke in parables and painted word pictures in His teachings. The understanding of calling Jesus 'Lord' was taught with images of building a house. "*But why do you call Me 'Lord, Lord,' and do not do the things which I say? Whoever comes to Me, and hears My sayings and does them, I will show you whom he is like: He is like a man building a house who dug deep and laid the foundation on the rock. And when the flood arose, the stream beat vehemently against that house, and could not shake it, for it was founded on the rock. But he who heard and did nothing is like a man who built a house on the earth without a foundation, against which the stream beat vehemently: and immediately it fell. And the ruin of that house was great"* (Luke 6:46-49). Isn't that easy to understand? Either we build our lives on the solid Rock, Christ Jesus and stand, or we build it on the sand (something else) and it falls.

Pictures help us to organize thoughts in our minds. Pictures give volumes of information and help us store information. A perfect illustration of this took place on Mother's Day in our church. Each Mother received a little gift bag and in it were items the pastor used to illustrate his message. Some of those items were a rubber band to remind us to be flexible, a band aid to remind us to take care of our children's hurts, a pencil to remind us to write down our blessings, an eraser to remind us to forget offences, a toothpick to remind us not to pick out people's faults, and candy hugs and kisses to remind us to give lots of hugs and kisses to our family. He cleverly painted pictures in our minds with images that mothers will remember for a long time.

As I pray for my son, I picture him playing his guitar in worship; I picture his leadership with teenagers and his radical love for Jesus. Many evangelists use the imaging technique by teaching the audience how to picture themselves:

1) See yourself set free (of drugs, alcohol, etc.)
2) See yourself living in victory
3) See yourself well, rather than sick
4) See yourself out of debt

Following the instruction in one imaging class, I asked the Holy Spirit to show me any problem areas in my life. I saw fear flashing like it was on a screen. Tears ran down my face because I felt so guilty. In my thinking, a believer should not have fear.

After asking me some questions, the instructor recommended I visit with one of the psychologists.

Since I had visited with Dr. Wakefield first, I went back to him. He pointed out that I was beating myself up. We discussed Rom 12:2 "*be transformed by the renewing of your mind…*" He asked me why there were verses in the Bible about fear? I assumed it was to show that we should never have fear; not realizing it was to help us get through our fear.

He continued, "What do you think about Peter walking on the water?"

I thought the lesson to be learned was, "It is wrong to fear."

He responded, "Is that all you get out of that story?" while he pointed out that it was a lesson where only one disciple had the courage to get out of the boat. Peter also knew whom to call out to when he started to sink. (Matthew 14:22-32) How skewed my thinking was on this issue. Dr. Wakefield discussed Jesus in the Garden of Gethsemane where He asked the Father three times, "*if it is possible, may this cup be taken from me*" (Matthew 26:42). Did Jesus have dread and fear what He was about to face? The Bible tells us He was human and tempted in every way as we are. Yes, He must have experienced fear in this situation. Even though His "*soul was overwhelmed with sorrow to the point of death*" (Matthew 26:38), He cried out, "Not my will but Thy will be done." In the midst of Jesus' darkest hour, He submitted to His Father with confidence.

Dr. Wakefield prayed that I would be free of fear, guilt, and doubts. Then he commented, "You carry more of the presence of God than any patient I've every had."

Emphatically I replied, "You have got to be kidding!"

He replied, "No, I am not."

In my room, I asked the Lord, "Why don't I feel the presence that he says he senses?" Obviously, more pruning was taking place. "Lord, I must trust You are with me, even when I am not 'feeling' like You are." It isn't wise to trust feelings, is it? They can lie to us, or deceive us, or destroy us. Feelings can lead to false pride, or they can lead to false condemnation, and I could easily identify with that.

On September 22, I had an appointment with the radiologist who was also studying my tests. He could not believe I was told to take no vitamins during the last series of radiation. This doctor stressed having good nutrition and vitamins. Neither could he understand why the radiologist in Missouri told me to wait a year for a checkup following the radiation, because the tumor should have been discovered sooner. Both doctors said there was enough evidence in the reports from Missouri of this cancer potentially happening. They could not understand why I was never given CT Scans to follow the situation.

Heidi, a young woman who was a teenager in the church we pastored several years ago, lives in Tulsa. She graciously invited us to her home for dinner one night; she took me for a tour of Tulsa and ORU and also brought me books, phone cards, and personal items. These were special times of renewing friendship and fellowship intermingled with all the tests and treatment. Her mother and sister came by my room to visit, too.

On September 26, the tumor board met at noon to study my test results. This board meets for critical cases, and together they would decide the best approach to deal with the situation. I asked the Lord to give them wisdom beyond their understanding. In my room I was listening to a CD with Scripture music. The following verse ministered so much: "*You are my servant, I have chosen you and have not cast you away: Fear not, for I am with you; be not dismayed, for I am your God. I will strengthen you, Yes, I will help you, I will uphold you with My righteous right hand*" (Isaiah 41:9b-10).

I had to hear the decision of the tumor board alone, because Arvy had gone back to Mayo Clinic for more appointments. The Lord prepared me with this word before the appointment with the surgeon. "*When you pass through the waters, I will be with you; and through the rivers, they shall not overflow you. When you walk through the fire, you shall not be burned, nor shall the flame scorch you. For I am the Lord your God, the Holy One of*

Israel, your Savior" (Isaiah 43:2-3a). Up to this point, I was very hesitant to have radiation again and dreaded it. From past experience and the previous radiologist's observations following the first series, I was well aware that my body did not handle radiation well. I wrote in my journal, "I will be told to have radiation." Nevertheless, the Scriptures prepared me, and the Lord removed the dread.

The board agreed that I should have four weeks of radiation, two weeks of IMRT radiation, and some chemotherapy. Radiation is a very specialized treatment program, which uses high-energy radiation beams. These procedures began the following day. During the twice-a-day treatments I recited the Scriptures like I had the first time.

Within a week I was having awful nausea because the radiation was also splashing onto my stomach. Following another imaging class, Dr. Ellison suggested an hour session with him to work on the nausea. He asked the Lord for the right images to be planted within me. After relaxing and continuing to ask the Holy Spirit's help, he quietly suggested images such as: see tasty food, imagine good food smells, visualize a calm stomach, picture smooth eating with no gagging. It worked. Praise the Lord!

While waiting at his appointment desk, I read a portion of an official document by a group of psychiatrists studying the "power of healing in the words we say to ourselves." Their research proves the impact of a patient speaking words of healing, and they are implementing that into their practice. Wow! That is scriptural and it has been God's plan all along His word states: *"Death and life are in the power of the tongue, and those who love it will eat its fruit"* (Proverbs 18:21). *"A wholesome tongue is a tree of life (health)…"* (Proverbs 14:4a). God has set spiritual laws into existence, and His laws are powerful and creative. If my words are not words of life, then they are words of death. If I'm not speaking victory, then I'm bound for defeat. Jesus said, *"For by your words you will be justified, and by your words you will be condemned.*" (Matthew 12:37)

Peter denied Jesus three times before His death. After His resurrection, Jesus asked Peter three times: "Peter, do you love Me?" Do you suppose Jesus wanted Peter to break or counterbalance the power of his negative words by having him speak positive words? "*There are those who speak rashly like the piercing of a sword, but the tongue of the wise brings healing*" (Proverbs 12:18, Amplified).

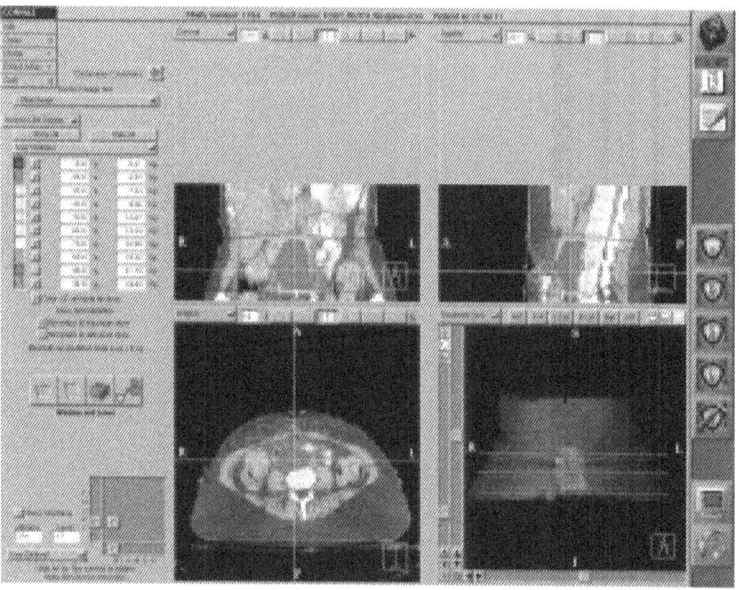

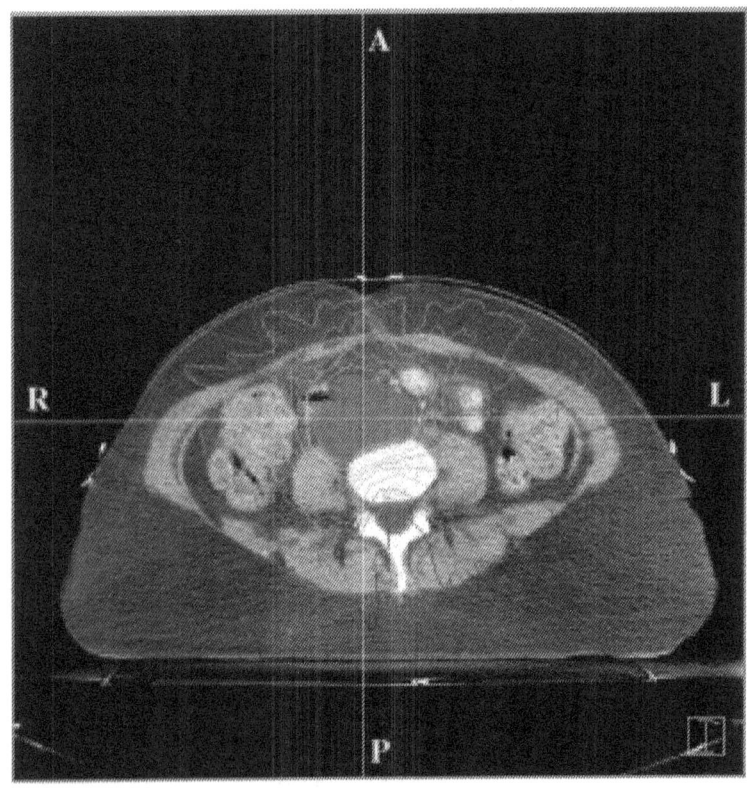

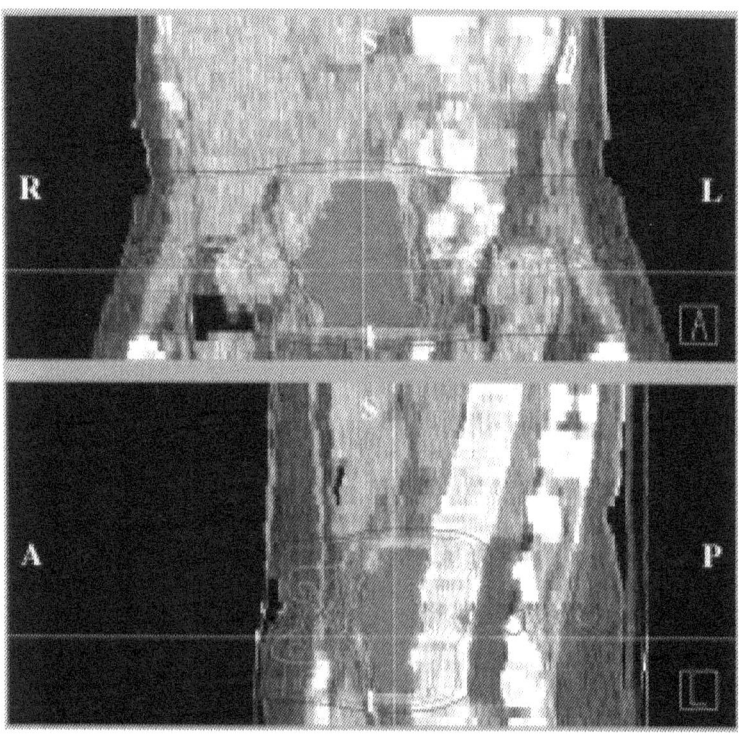

Charged Up Like a Battery

Chapter 7

The nausea stopped after the imaging session, but intense vomiting continued for about four weeks. With the nausea gone, I had no clue when I would vomit. With no warning, I vomited the entire evening meal onto the dinner tray just as I finished eating. I was so embarrassed, even though other patients rushed to my aid, took the tray, and cleaned up the mess. The next evening it happened again. Following those two episodes I carried a container everywhere I went. Also, food so repulsed my stomach, that I simply warmed up a cup of soup in a microwave and ate it in my room or ate only a little paper cup of sherbet for many days.

That Sunday morning was spent in the lab area because I was running a fever after the first week of radiation. Blood cultures were taken and five times they tried to get an IV started since my body was getting dehydrated. The promise from Psalm 57:1b-2 gave me strength and encouragement: "*For my soul trusts in You; and in the shadow of Your wings I will make my refuge, until these calamities have passed by. I will cry out to God Most High, to God who performs all things for me.*" The next day in a one-hour surgery, the surgeon put a port in my chest. That made a way for IV's, blood input, infusion of anti-vomiting medication twice daily, and chemotherapy sessions without having to use the veins in my arms. I was so glad to get the anti-vomiting medication through the port because it worked better. No longer did I have to cope with swallowing a pill and it coming right back up. Also, Medicare covered the cost of the injections, but I had to purchase the pills. The pills were $42 each and one prescription cost $365; financially it was impossible for me to purchase more. My red blood count went too low, resulting in a night spent in the infusion department with two units of blood administered.

Some visitors during this time later told me they thought I was dying. Near the end of October, the psychologist Dr. Ellison called me in my room. While praying for me, he sensed the Lord wanted to convey a message to me. He encouraged me to pray in tongues every day and have someone pray with me every day in tongues. I was so weak that I could only pray a few words at a time. The apostle Paul states, "*I thank my God I speak with tongues more than you all*" (I Corinthians 14:18). Why did Paul say that? The only gift listed for personal edification is tongues; and Paul explains that when we speak in an unknown tongue, we are "edified" or "charged". (I Corinthians 14:4) A rephrase of this verse might be, "He who speaks in a tongue charges himself up like a battery"; therefore, it is a supernatural means of building up our spiritual life.

In verse 14 of the same chapter, Paul explains that praying in a tongue is the spirit praying. Even Jesus stated that this sign would follow those who believe in Mark 16:17. I needed all the indwelling presence of the Holy Spirit to survive. I wasn't sure how to pray specifically in the situation, but the Bible says the Spirit makes intercession for us according to the will of the Father. "*Likewise the Spirit also helps in our weaknesses. For we do not know what we should pray for as we ought, but the Spirit Himself makes intercession for us...He makes intercession for the saints according to the will of God*" (Romans 8:26-27). When in the midst of turmoil, perplexity, or anxiety, praying in tongues stimulates faith. "*But you, beloved, building yourselves up on your most holy faith, praying in the Holy Spirit*" (Jude 20).

Praying or singing in the Spirit does not heal us, but it helps us to trust the Lord more fully because it charges our faith. Even Isaiah writes about the refreshing and rest to the weary when speaking in this manner. (28:11-12) How I needed spiritual and physical refreshing! As I became stronger, I was able to sing in the spirit as well; and Paul explains that praying and singing in the Spirit "*gives thanks well.*" (I Corinthians 14:15-17) I like to call this devotional praying and singing in the Spirit, for in public meetings it is better to speak words of understanding, according to Paul's directions. (I Corinthians 14:18-19)

The same week I received a letter stating, "I feel like the Lord is saying get four to five people to pray and sing in the Spirit for a half hour over you." I didn't know how to gather a group together in Tulsa, but Mary called a group together in Mason City to pray. Afterwards, Helen called a friend in Tulsa who came with a group, and they prayed with me for over an hour. Victory Christian Center sent people two to three times a week to call upon the Lord with me. My home church and many all over the country were interceding as relatives and friends requested prayer. My husband could see something in my eyes that indicated a slight change for the better after the hour-long prayer time.

Within a short time, the nutritionist intervened, and I was given nutritional IV's for several days. Those gave me strength enough to start eating a few bites each meal. At the same time I had finished the four weeks of radiation and was being prepared for the Intensity Modulated Radiation Therapy (IMRT). With IMRT the therapist can treat difficult-to-reach tumors with new levels of accuracy. They are able to use radiation doses up to 40 percent higher than traditional methods would allow in these areas. IMRT directs radiation at the tumor and modulates the intensity of pencil-thin beams of radiation with laser accuracy.

The recipient is fitted with a plastic cast by putting very warm plastic over the body from the neck to the thighs. The plastic is molded into a skin-tight form that will be placed over the person and bolted onto a table in eight places when the IMRT is administered. This is to keep the body from moving during the intense radiation, which takes more than a half hour each day. With the use of a CT scan, markings were placed on the plastic form while I lay under it, because treatments had to be done with extreme precision.

I had to deal with intense apprehension and nervousness before the IMRT procedures began. Perhaps it was a type of phobia. The thought of being bolted to a table for about 45 minutes per treatment seemed insurmountable. What if I vomited? What if I had to go to the bathroom? How am I going to get through this? The Friday before they were to begin, a beautiful homemade card came with the same Scripture the Lord had given me about radiation four weeks earlier. The next day another letter arrived stating the same Scripture in Isaiah 43:2-3: *"When you pass through the waters, I will be with you; and through the rivers, they shall not overflow you. When you walk through the fire, you shall not be burned, nor shall the flames scorch you. For I am the Lord your God, the Holy One of Israel, your Savior."* The Lord is so good to bring comfort, and He used two people to remind me of His promise. During the same weekend, the Lord quickened the following verses to me: *"For You, O God, have proved us; You have refined us as silver is refined. You brought us into the net; You laid affliction on our backs. You have caused men to ride over our heads; we went through fire and through water; but You brought us out to rich fulfillment"* (Psalm 66:10-12). Yes! Hallelujah!

The IMRT personnel allowed me to wear earphones to listen to a CD with Scripture songs during the daily procedure. I have learned in the depth of pain, weakness, and the unknown that filling the mind with Scripture is vitally important, for it brings life in the midst of difficult situations. Psalm 119 has many verses describing what the Word will do in a person's life.

Phone calls from relatives and friends were the highlight of the day, plus the cards and mail. Helen used a different approach with her phone calls. She helped me to laugh. The Bible says, "*Laughter is good medicine.*" Meanwhile, an unusual card arrived with the face of a bulldog on the front. Inside were these words, "Sorry you are having such a poopy day." When Helen called on days I was very sick and weak from vomiting, my first response would be, "This is one of those super poopy days." She understood, and we laughed heartily. Humor classes are held at the center every week, because it has been proven laughter releases endorphins that help with the emotions, pain, and healing of the body.

My daughter, Nancy, flew in for a weekend. That was a blessed break from the routine of radiation. Her husband, Dave, came by to visit twice when he had business in Tulsa. Arvy was in and out for a week or two at time between his visits to the Mayo Clinic where they were continuing to get him stabilized with his diabetes and potassium levels.

A lady walked up to me the first week at the Cancer Treatment Center and said, "Ruth, you have given and given and given throughout your life. The Lord has shown me that He wants you to receive and receive and receive." What a surprise! She didn't even know me. The Lord provided many prayer warriors, encouragers, and finances. Several times throughout the ten-week process, a letter would come with money and those finances helped pay some of the room charges. Thank you Lord for all your obedient children. God is faithful and so good!

Master of Breakthroughs

Chapter 8

People were coming by my room nearly every day to pray with me. It is amazing to sense the love and concern of others; truly it is a picture of the body of Christ functioning as He would desire. I commend the faithful volunteers from Victory Christian Center who came several times each week to pray. Nurses, doctors, and personnel at the cancer center, and others all over the United States prayed for me as well.

I was released to go home about a week before Thanksgiving on a very cold morning. Helen and her sister Mary came to Tulsa to drive me home. As we were nearing Des Moines, word came over the radio that the city had extremely icy roads, and the freeways were blocked with accidents. We stopped in a little town for the night. While driving to find a place to eat, we saw an attractive display of Christmas lights in the town square. What a cultural shock! When I entered the cancer center it was 105 degrees; now it was cold and windy, plus Christmas decorations were displayed. I had been gone over ten weeks.

After getting home, I went to my drawers and closets to get clothes, and they were filled with summer clothes. I had to get my winter clothes out and exchange them for the summer clothes. That made reality set in quickly.

The next few weeks were a flurry of activity. Holidays are always full and extremely happy. Mary had Thanksgiving and Christmas dinners. I was unable to do the cooking, and I was having difficulty eating. Nevertheless, it was especially good for me to be with the family. I was extremely aware how much everyone meant to me, especially this Christmas. I had to lie down for awhile, but I spent every minute I could with the family, even though it was extremely exhausting. It was hard to contain tears of joy for the privilege of being with them.

I was seriously struggling with the challenge Dr. Ellison gave me before going home. He asked, "On a scale of one to ten, where do you stand in believing you are healed?" I couldn't answer that. He wrote notes on my case as he was searching for keys and better ways of working or praying with people to be healed. I wasn't feeling victorious. I felt poor and needy. My body was thin and gaunt. I prayed, "*Save me according to your love, Lord.*" "*This is my comfort in my affliction, for Your word has given me life*" (Psalm 119:50). I hung onto the promise: "*I shall not die, but live, and declare the works of the Lord*" (Psalm 118:17). The struggle for the answer to Dr. Ellison's question haunted me. Finally, I realized my life and spirit were full of the Word, and Jesus sends His Word and heals us. There was nothing else to do but rely on Jesus, no matter what the outcome.

Time was quickly slipping by and my next appointment was January 7. I was trying to pray, to confess, to believe, and one day I felt worn out calling for help. "*I am weary with my crying; my throat is dry; my eyes fail while I wait for my God*" (Psalm 69:3). I believe the Lord was continuing to call others to do battle for me. About a week before returning to Tulsa, the Lord spoke to my heart to write down every phrase in the book of Psalm that expressed who He is. Here are some examples from those seven pages:

> *"The Lord remains faithful forever."*
> *"Great is our Lord and mighty in power."*
> *"The Lord's unfailing love surrounds the man who trusts in Him."*
> *"The Lord is my rock, my fortress, and my deliverer."*

"The Lord is the one who sustains me."
"You are awesome, O God."
"You are the God who performs miracles."
"The Lord's great love is forever."
"Rest in the shadow of the Almighty."
"The faithfulness of the Lord endures forever."

A newsletter from Mario Murillo arrived a few days before we were to go to the cancer center. He was discussing one of David's darkest moments turning to sudden light. He asked the question, "Is your spirit exhausted from warfare?"

I cried, "Yes." Then he quoted II Samuel 5:20 which says, "*So David went to Baal Perazim, and David defeated them there; and he said, "The Lord has broken through my enemies before me, like a breakthrough of water." Therefore he called the name of that place Baal Perazim.*" He explained that in David's first battle against the Philistines, God's deliverance came like a flash flood. David was so stunned that he named the place of victory Baal Perazim, which literally means Master of Breakthroughs. He also said that 90 percent of any crisis is the fear generated by the crisis, not the circumstances themselves; and fear is defeated when you know that the battle is the Lord's.

A ray of sunshine burst upon my soul, because I knew the battle was the Lord's. My God is the Master of Breakthroughs! The inspiration from the newsletter and the phrases from the Psalms greatly lifted my spirit. I felt renewed, optimistic, and hopeful for a good report. I did not know for certain that I was healed or that the report would say the cancer was gone. The Lord had filled me to overflowing with the Word, and I could trust Him in all things. Maybe that takes more faith than making a statement that I know I am healed. "*Now faith is the substance of things hoped for, the evidence of things not seen*" (Hebrews 11:1). At last, I could face going back to the cancer center.

The Lord promises us peace when our mind is fixed on Him. He will keep us in perfect peace when we keep our mind steadfast on Him, and always trust Him because He is the Rock we can always stand on. (See Isaiah 26:3-4) Searching the Scriptures, reading them, and listening to Scripture songs transforms a person's thinking. Negative thinking cannot remain. Negative thoughts are opposite the Lord's thoughts. *"You will guard him and keep him in perfect and constant peace whose mind [both its inclination and its character] is stayed on You, because he commits himself to You, leans on You, and hopes confidently in You. So trust in the Lord—commit yourself to Him, lean on Him, hope confidently in Him—for ever; for the Lord God is an everlasting rock—the rock of ages"* (Isaiah 26:2-3, Amplified).

On January 8, a bone scan and a CT scan were done to locate the tumor so that the physician could make the necessary decisions for further procedures. The next day I would receive the verdict. When the doctor walked in, he said, "I have a good report. We cannot see any cancer, but there is scar tissue." He felt I needed six months of preventative chemo as a precaution. However, he said that I was too weak and too thin to begin immediately; instead, he asked me to come back in February. He gave me a big hug.

It was with tremendous joy that I went to all the departments and shared the good news and received hugs from everyone. As one nurse hugged me she commented, "This is a God miracle."

Highly Lethal Condition

Chapter 9

Two days after arriving home from the Cancer Treatment Center, our pastor was happy to announce that the cancer was gone, and he called me a "trophy of the faith." During Sunday School the teacher prayed for me. Then he shared a word from the Lord, "Ruth, the Lord is not done with you yet." While driving back to church that evening, I became very ill, and we had to return home. Before reaching home, I cried out, "Stop," and I opened the door and vomited. An hour later I vomited about a quart of blood and passed out. My husband helped me up off the bathroom floor, and I passed more blood in the stool. He called 911. The ambulance rushed me to the hospital with IV's and oxygen started.

X-rays were taken immediately, a tube was put through the nose to the stomach to pump out the blood, and a unit of blood was started. Arvy, Mary, and Pastor Close stayed with me until about midnight. Pastor felt that the enemy was trying to steal the Lord's trophy. At 4 a.m. the nurse called Arvy back to the hospital as I was in systemic shock—no blood pressure. When I came to I heard the nurses discuss the dangerous situation after they got the blood pressure up to 50/20; two units of blood were under pressure to enter the body quickly and 1500 cc was going through the IV every hour. Later a camera was put into my stomach to check for a bleeding ulcer, but that was not the problem. Due to the urgency of sustaining my life, a CT Scan was taken with the use of an IV dye to get detailed diagnostic information about the loss of blood. The CT Scan revealed a blown aorta that was spurting into the small intestine.

The surgeon told the family that I was in a lethal condition. He offered the following facts: "without surgery her chances are 100 percent fatal, with surgery it is 90 percent fatal (Mayo cardiology department says 99 percent fatal). If the surgery is successful, there are serious problems that can develop: (1) If the shunt fails, the body parts that it supplies will have to be amputated. (2) If the surgery is successful, there is danger of kidney failure, liver failure, and complications with the lungs." The surgeon also stated that if he was back to see the family within 15 minutes, surgery was unsuccessful. He felt the surgery should take about 3½ hours. When those in the waiting room hadn't heard anything for 4½ hours, Arvy was emotionally preparing to face the possibility that a leg had to be amputated. Before surgery 7 units of blood were pumped into my body, during surgery 12 more units of blood were given, and following surgery 4 additional units were administered.

During the surgery family and friends were called to pray. Four and one half hours later the family was told that the surgery was successful, but that the next few days would be critical as far as complications developing; and my chance for recovery was 50-50. The family and pastor commented that they had prayed during surgery, and the surgeon said that he had prayed for himself, too. He also explained that I would be under immobilization drugs for a few days and morphine for pain.

I was out of it for six days, except for a few very brief periods. I remember once knowing my daughter Sheryl was in the room, and she told me she loved me, and I was out again. The seventh morning I was awake enough to know my daughter Nancy was there. However, with the ventilator still breathing for me, I could not talk. That was a bit frustrating, as I couldn't respond to her visiting, but it was so comforting to see her. That day I learned that the hospital doctors, nurses, and personnel were calling me the "miracle lady on 6th floor", which is the critical care unit. Even though still very ill, I knew God's hand was upon me and that many were praying for me. As the family came in from day to day, the nurses would comment, "She is doing really good," but then they always warned that serious complications could still develop.

One precious lady from the church came in to my room and said, "Well done, good and faithful servant." Those short words ministered remarkable life and encouragement to me. Then she told me that the Lord spoke to her to come into the room each day and whisper that into my ear, even when I was unconscious. Mary, my daughter, also brought a CD player and kept Scripture music playing.

Once I was fully awake, the surgeon told me some of what he had to do in the surgery. He explained that the scar tissue from the radiation had infused the aorta into the small intestine, which caused the aorta to blow a hole. He had to sew up the aorta. He also had to remove the second and third portion of the duodenum and six inches of the small intestine. There was no blood reaching the right leg, so a left-to-right shunt (bypass) was performed to get the circulation to the right leg. Interestingly, he did not see any evidence of a tumor, though visualization of the abdominal area was difficult because of the radiation fibrosis. He commented that I had gone through a very invasive surgery and that it would take a lot of time to recover.

On the tenth day, the ventilator was removed, and I started breathing on my own. The vocal chords were so damaged or bruised by the ventilator, I could only whisper. It took about eight weeks to get my speaking voice and about fifteen weeks before I was able to sing. The following day I was released from the critical care unit and taken to the surgical floor. Two therapists helped me begin to walk a little each day, and a few days later the stomach tube was removed, and I was given a liquid diet.

The surgeon warned me that I would be a little puky for a while because of the way the intestine was now hooked onto the stomach. As soon as I was given food, I started vomiting which continued for several days. One evening the surgeon told me that if the vomiting didn't stop the next day, he would have to put tubes back into the stomach and go back to intravenous feeding. Out of desperation, I called the church and asked for everyone to pray, as there were services that evening. From depths of my being burst an anguished cry, "Oh, God, please stop the vomiting now, in the name of Jesus Christ my Lord." The vomiting stopped immediately. Another answer to prayer! Two days later I was released to go home after nineteen days in the hospital.

I wondered if I could make it into our home, because of incredible loss of strength. Arvy had to do everything; he cooked, cleaned, washed clothes, and took care of me. Two weeks after the release from the hospital, the surgeon wanted to see me (five weeks after surgery). It was a huge undertaking to go for an appointment, because of unbelievable weakness. It took every bit of will power I could muster to dress, get into the car, and somehow walk to his office. At that time he was quite concerned because the shunt was not working properly. I asked him what he could do if the shunt did not begin working properly? He didn't know for sure what could be done. That was a little scary, because it could lead to amputation. As long as I was still weak and quiet, he felt there was nothing to worry about. He scheduled me to see him again in five weeks.

The first time I attended church was the Sunday before that next appointment. The pastor was unaware of my latest situation, but the Lord led him to open the altar in the middle of the song service for people to come to be anointed with oil and prayed over for healing. *"Is anyone among you sick? Let him call for the elders of the church, and let them pray over him, anointing him with oil in the name of the Lord. And the prayer of faith will save the sick, and the Lord will raise him up"* (James 5:14-15a). I went forward, and the pastor interceded for me. As the surgeon examined me this time, he lit up like a light bulb. Several times he said, "Great, the shunt is working" as he took the pulse up and down the leg. Four weeks later he checked the circulation and shunt again, and it was working fine. WOW!

Praise the Lord! Another answer to prayer! I gained a new appreciation for the anointing oil as I read the verse from Isaiah 10:27: "*It shall come to pass in that day that his burden will be taken away from your shoulder, and his yoke from your neck, and the yoke will be destroyed because of the anointing oil.*" Yes, the yoke was destroyed!

Eating was one of the most difficult lingering problems to deal with after arriving home. My stomach was still shrunk from the radiation experience when nothing would stay down and very little was eaten. The aftereffects of radiation kept my stomach irritated and caused it to be upset easily. Added to that was the time in the hospital with no food. The nurse described my stomach as about the size of a lemon. Many times food or the smell of it would repulse me, or cause me to gag, or just taste awful. Now, I could identify with an anorexic person.

About eight weeks after surgery I weighed, and to my amazement, the scale said 111 pounds. Because of the nutritional training at the cancer center, I knew the amount of weight loss was critical and that I was malnourished. My stomach was only able to take a half to one cup of food—usually soup—at a time, and eating three times a day was not enough nourishment. Immediately, I forced myself to sip protein drinks: between breakfast and lunch I drank a soy protein drink with juice, and mid-afternoon I drank a sport protein drink with raspberries, bananas, milk, and cream added. Two weeks later, a pound of weight had been added. It was an uphill battle for several months, but the protein began to build up my body, resulting in a little strength returning. Getting well was such a long process; it seemed I would never be in good physical health again. Fifteen weeks after surgery, my stomach began to accept more food and it had fewer upsets. I was beginning to gain weight, and strength began returning at a quicker pace. Finally, I was able to help some with the cooking and washing clothes.

The doctor of internal medicine has also been keeping tabs on me. During the first visit with him, he commented, "You are an answer to prayer. Hallelujah!" What a surprise. To hear a doctor say that is indeed remarkable. I was so excited, that I asked if he wanted to hear about another miracle, and he replied, "Yes." Quickly I told him about praying for the shunt to work properly, and he responded, "God does answer prayer." Truly, I am amazed to be alive!

While I was in the hospital, they used my port for IV's. Now it was time to have it accessed, or as they say, "flushed." I had to go to the lab at the cancer center to get it done because the port is supposed to be flushed every 30 days. This will be an ongoing process until it is time to have the port removed.

The Nightmare

Chapter 10

When the gynecologist diagnosed the cancer of the uterus lining, he explained that it was hormonally induced, and he warned me to never take estrogen again. The memories of a bad experience in another state a few years ago came flooding back.

One summer I was spotting a lot until it turned into hemorrhaging. Quickly I got an appointment with my gynecologist. Immediately upon examination, he determined that I needed a D&C. As I explained to him our insurance situation had changed to an HMO, he felt they would certainly proceed with the same recommendation. The cost to have him do the out patient surgery was more than we could afford.

The HMO was a totally different situation (in those days). It seemed they would do anything to prevent surgical procedures from taking place. Slowly across a two-month time frame, they did test after test, such as an ultra sound, x-rays, blood tests, and a biopsy. A week or more lapsed between each test. Finally, when the biopsy was done, I talked with the doctor about my concerns of this dragging on and on and nothing being done. She assured me she was there to get this resolved, that I would know within seven days the results of the biopsy and whether or not a D&C would be performed, and she suggested I call the clinic to get the results.

Now the nightmare began. I started calling, and they kept giving me a run around. When I asked for the doctor by name, she was never in. When I asked about the test results, several different answers were given: (1) the tests aren't back, (2) we can't find your tests results, (3) the test was lost—after I had been told the results were back, (4) or the person speaking didn't have the authority to give me the results. This went on for 3½ weeks until my sister arrived from out of state. She was disturbed by my condition and boldly called the clinic. First she was told that the doctor that did the biopsy did not work there but only filled in for a couple of days. After enduring the run around from several different rude personnel, she demanded to speak to the manager. She explained the situation and angrily demanded action. Finally, after several hours of intense phone calls, the clinic asked me to go to the emergency room at one of the hospitals where their head gynecologist was working that day.

I asked my daughter to go along and to sit in the examination room as my witness. By this time, I was made to feel that it was all in my head and that I was some kind of a mental nut. Even though bleeding is not "in the head," emotionally I was a basket case.

After the examination and the explanation of the run around from the clinic, the doctor's diagnosis was that I did not need a D&C. First, he prescribed a week of medication to cause this collection of cells on the uterine wall to hopefully bleed out. Then he doubled my prescription for hormones, telling me this would stop all periods, and everything would be great from then on.

Can you imagine the horror in January 1999 of hearing the cancer was hormonally induced and realizing the HMO doctor in another state had done me a great injustice? The only choice I had was to forgive him. If I wanted the Lord to be with me and help me through this, I needed His grace, mercy, and love. *"For if you forgive people their trespass—that is, their reckless and willful sins, leaving them, letting them go and giving up resentment—your heavenly Father will also forgive you. But if you do not forgive others their trespasses—their reckless and willful sins, leaving them, letting them go and giving up resentment—neither will your Father forgive you your trespasses"* (Matthew 6:14-15, Amplified). If we meet certain conditions, there is no limitation to Jesus Christ's law of forgiveness. The conditions are repentance and confession.

At the Cancer Treatment Center of America two doctors from different departments stated that I did not have the follow up after surgery and radiation that I should have had in the previous cancer facility in another state. The tumor should have been caught much sooner. Does one forgive or get bitter? I chose to forgive; I certainly didn't have the time or strength to waste on bitterness, and I needed every bit of God's power and stamina to face this ordeal.

A new circumstance faced me after arriving home from the ten weeks in Tulsa. Friends and family were understandably distraught and frustrated over what I had been through and was still experiencing. Several pressed me to sue the previous doctors, and they located a lawyer that works on commission only. A highly trained medical person explained that suing was not for my benefit, but to put a stop to medical practices that are not right. I pondered that and understood the implications but continued to be uneasy about it. Since I knew I had forgiven them, how could I sue?

Shortly thereafter, the aorta blew and the whole hospital episode took place with the words echoing in my ears, "Miracle lady on 6th floor;" such a remarkable peace enveloped me. The answer was obvious. God has seen me through so much, He is so good, He spared my life, He is the Master of Breakthroughs, and He is all-powerful. Why would I even consider suing mere man?

Ruth E. Foat

Greatly Enlarged In Him

Chapter 11

Our pastor preached two messages with reference to the prayer of Jabez taken from I Chronicles 4:10: "*And Jabez called on the God of Israel saying, "Oh, that You would bless me indeed, and enlarge my territory, that Your hand would be with me, and that You would keep me from evil, that I may not cause pain!" So God granted him what he requested.*" The NIV translation changes the last phrase slightly, "that I may be free of pain." He shared with us how important this prayer must have been because a line of genealogy is interrupted to include the prayer.

Jabez's name means sorrow maker. In the Old Testament, names given to people identified the character-type of the person. Such as Judah means praise. Many times when the Israelites went to war, the tribe of Judah was in the lead to praise the Lord in the midst of battle. One story told in II Chronicles 20 shows the great victory God provided with singers and praise leading them into battle. Understanding the importance of one's name in Hebrew thinking helps us to comprehend Jabez's difficult situation. God honored his prayer and apparently he was raised above the blight of his name.

Jabez's prayer seems so effortless, and it almost sounds self-centered to pray for personal blessing. God wants to impart supernatural favor and goodness upon us, but He wants us to ask for it. The Lord's blessings are not for personal gain, but for our territory to be enlarged. God wants to bring more opportunities and people across our paths to whom He can minister His grace.

We will need His ability and strength to accomplish ministry in that greater territory; therefore, we need the "*Lord's hand with us,*" lest we become weary and faint.

The phrase, "*You would keep me from evil,*" has taken on special significance to me. Because of the many miracles in my life the last two years, I don't want to rely on past victories nor to become complacent. Rather I see the need for more supernatural help to protect me from Satan's ability to tempt me or to have a false view of my strengths. These experiences have caused me to rely on the Lord more. During radiation treatments, The Lord's Prayer was always part of my prayer. The phrase "*lead us not into temptation, but deliver us from the evil one*," (Matthew 6:13a) agrees with Jabez's prayer "*keep me from evil.*" Since Jesus was teaching the crowds how to pray, this has to be an important part of prayer. I would rather be kept from the evil one, than to be caught in the middle of temptation.

Our Pastor challenged us to pray Jabez's prayer for thirty days. Testimonies are coming forth with some unusual answers to the prayer. In view of the fact that pain was quite prevalent in my body, I chose to pray the last phrase from two different translations: "*that I may not cause pain and that I will be free from pain.*" I continued to pray the same prayer after the 30 days. The intriguing facet is that the pain is less in my thigh bursa area, which started as a result of inflammation from radiation two years ago. The Lord is continuing to answer prayer, and I plan to continue this prayer daily. This prayer has also become part of my prayer for my pastor, for my children, and for others as the Lord directs.

Job trusted God in the midst of great sorrow and pain (Job 2:13) even though his wife was telling him to "curse God and die." His despair was so overwhelming, he longed to die and Job said, "*Though He slay me, yet I will trust Him*" (Job 13:15). The thief comes to steal, kill, and destroy (John 10:10). Though Satan is the destroyer, the Lord sovereignly uses our trials to draw us into a deeper relationship with him. We may be tested by fire and pruned severely. Even Jesus learned obedience through the things He suffered (Hebrews 5:8-9). Suffering isn't an option! It may not be physical suffering, but some type of pressure must come so that we learn to overcome (Revelation 12:11).

I've faced several life-threatening situations: surgery after surgery and cancer after cancer—and as a needy person I sought physical healing as well as spiritual strength. While I trusted Him in the midst of suffering, I never gave up my confidence in the Lord. Not only has my body been healed, but also my spirit and soul have been greatly enlarged in Him.

In these latter days, I sense the Lord is preparing us to stand; this remnant will be stretched, tested, tried, and proven. Self-pity will flow out of us if we have our eyes on the dealings of the Lord, rather than on the Lord who is doing the dealing. The disciples asked Jesus, "*What will be the sign of your coming?*" Jesus responded that some will be deceived, some will be killed; there will be famines, pestilence, and earthquakes; many will be offended, "*But he who endures to the end shall be saved*" (Matthew 24:4-14).

There are so many heavy things going on today: divorce, abuse, violence, predators, bullying, uprisings, ethnic cleansings, terrorists, persecution; plus pressures financially, emotionally, physically, and relationally. The Lord is toughening us up! He is not interested in a mamby pamby feel-good religion. He is after a radical sold-out believer who is willing to pay the price to follow Him through anything, who is passionately in love with Him, who is full of the joy of the Lord, and who will choose to rejoice in Him in the midst of hardships and scarcity. "*Though the fig tree does not blossom, and there be no fruit on the vines; [though] the product of the olive fail, and the fields yield no food; though the flock be cut off from the fold, and there be no cattle in the stalls; yet I will rejoice in the Lord, I will exult in the [victorious] God of my salvation! The Lord God is my strength, my personal bravery and my invincible army; He makes my feet like hinds' feet, and will make me to walk [not to stand still in terror, but to walk] and make [spiritual] progress upon my high places [of trouble, suffering or responsibility]* (Habbakkuk 3:17-19, Amplified)! Hallelujah!

Some believers want Jesus for the benefits they receive, rather than serving Him as our Lord and King. The three Hebrew children, Shadrach, Meshach, and Abed-Nego were ordered by a sneering King Nebuchadnezzar to be cast into a burning furnace. "*Who will deliver you from my hands*" (Daniel 3:15)? What a classic response they gave, "*If that is the case, our God whom we serve is able to deliver us from the burning fiery furnace, and He will deliver us from your hand, O king. But if not, let it be known to you, O king, that we do not serve your gods, nor will we worship the gold image which you have set up*" (Daniel 3:17-18).

Jesus knew there would be rough times ahead for He instructed the people to "*Come to Me, all you who labor and are heavy laden, and I will give you rest.*" As we give Him our burdens and take on His easy yoke, "*the people who know their God shall be strong and carry out great exploits*" (Daniel 11:32). This remnant will learn the joy of the Lord is their strength, and laughter will release much tension and despair.

Why?

Chapter 12

One day while visiting in the hospital, my pastor commented about the two great miracles that had recently taken place in my body. First, the cancerous mass was gone and secondly, I had recovered from a lethal condition with the aorta. My immediate response was, "I hope the Lord uses someone else for the next miracle. I can't handle anymore." Later I repented for that statement. I always want to be where the Lord can use me the most effectively. *"I have tested you in the furnace of affliction, for My own sake, for My own sake, I will do it; for how should My name be profaned? And I will not give My glory to another"* (Isaiah 48:10b-11).

However, a fleeting thought crossed my mind several times, "Why did I have to go through all this?" I felt that the enemy of my life was trying to steal, kill, and destroy me. I did not ask in anger nor did I blame God. But I would like to know if He had a purpose through it all.

Palm Sunday, our pastor was speaking about the Triumphal Entry of Jesus into Jerusalem. He was explaining that the Lord wanted us to praise him not only with our voices, but also with our "stuff." He told about the man that let Jesus use his donkey. He urged the congregation to let God use their stuff, such as their car or their home. A wrenching cry came from deep within, "Lord, You know I have done that in the past, but Lord I am so weak, what can I do now?" As he continued, the little chorus ran through my mind, "To be used of God, to sing, to pray…" At that moment, the Lord dropped a word into my heart, "You allowed me to use your body so that my name would be glorified at the hospital, among the doctors, nurses, and personnel." As tears came to my eyes, I whispered, "Thank you Jesus for helping me understand." When I shared this with Pastor Close, he commented, "That sounds like a living sacrifice." (Romans 12:1) It reminds me again of the phrase in Isaiah at the beginning of this chapter, "*I will not give My glory to another.*"

There is an account in the gospel of John about Jesus healing a man born blind. The disciples questioned Jesus about his blindness, "Was it the man's fault or his parent's fault?"

Jesus answered, "*It was not that this man or his parents sinned; but he was born blind in order that the workings of God should be manifested—displayed and illustrated—in him.*" (John 9:2, Amplified)

The Lord doesn't use angels to witness of His glory. He uses people. "*But you are a chosen generation, a royal priesthood, a holy nation, His own special people, that you may proclaim the praises of Him who called you out of darkness into His marvelous light*" (I Peter 2:9). God is looking for a people who will trust him before the whole world through impossible situations. He wants to present a faithful people who have been rocked by hard times, broken by deep trials, yet who continue to trust Him. He wants a people who will be shining examples of His grace and love. He wants this people to be at rest in their soul, because they know God is in control of everything concerning them.

One day I was talking with the Lord about the amazing fact that the hospital personnel called me "the miracle lady of 6th floor," and I was thanking Him for all who had prayed for me. I was sure I had nothing to do with it, when the Lord spoke to my heart again. He said, "But I prepared your spirit by asking you to write out the phrases from the Psalms and you were obedient." I want to be a soldier who is fully prepared for the battlefield. When the enemy comes at me suddenly, I want to be equipped. The powerful Word of God supplies that preparation, as I study and hide it away in my heart. So, the next time the enemy attacks, hopefully I will have reserves to draw on. I am convinced of His love only by devouring His Word and cultivating intimacy with Him through prayer.

The Lord completely amazes me as He unfolds His truth to us. *"When you pass through the waters, I will be with you; and through the rivers, they shall not overflow you. When you walk through the fire, you shall not be burned, nor shall the flame scorch you. For I am the Lord your God"* (Isaiah 43:2). When this promise was given to me at the cancer center, I did not realize a few verses later there was an explanation. *"Because you are precious in My sight, and honored, and I love you, I give men in return for you and peoples in exchange for your life"* (Isaiah 43:4, Amplified). The following verses describe the offspring He will bring back *"even every one who is called by My name, whom I have created for My glory, whom I have formed, whom I have made"* (Isaiah 43:7). What joy springs in my heart! What wonderful promises! Our God is so good to continually open His Word to His people. May He be glorified through my life!

Offense or Victory

Chapter 13

In the previous chapters I have woven threads of the Father's pruning—-an amazing plan to keep His children thriving physically, mentally, emotionally and spiritually. Little did I comprehend the depth of what lay ahead of me when the Lord spoke to my heart about the pruning He wanted to do even as I was cutting the raspberry canes off at the ground. This time of pruning has been more intense than ever before in my life. He knew my heart's desire to be conformed into His image, to produce more fruit, and to seek His kingdom first. If Jesus chose us for abundance and created us to deeply desire it, how can we ever find fulfillment in anything less?

On the night of Jesus betrayal, He spoke to His disciples about the true vine and the branches. The picture begins to unfold in John 14:31 as Jesus says, "*Come now; let us leave.*" They left the upper room and Jesus led them along the ancient vineyards as they headed to the Mount of Olives where the agony of Gethsemane began. In this setting Jesus calmly speaks about the grapes, the vines, and branches and how the gardener cares for his cherished vineyard. As Jesus portrays their future, it certainly isn't what they expect to hear. Jesus says, "*He (the gardener) cuts off every branch in me that bears no fruit, while every branch that does bear fruit he trims clean so that it will be even more fruitful*" (John 15:2 NIV).

I planted and pruned all kinds of fruit in Southern Missouri by following the instructions in several county extension bulletins. One of them included the growing and pruning of grapes and I learned several facts:

> Grapes tend to grow vigorously and a lot of the wood must be cut away every year. If the wood is not cut away, the vine will produce new luxurious growth but no grapes. Grapevines can become so thick that the sun cannot reach into the area where fruit should form. As the vine ages, the plant weakens and its crop decreases unless intense pruning is done; therefore, mature branches must be pruned relentlessly to receive the highest yields.

The Lord has been opening my understanding regarding another area so deep within that I didn't realize it was there. Apparently, I had arrived at the stage in my life where the branches were being pruned extensively to produce the best yields. The Lord's promise "I would not die, but live," kept me through the first series of radiation. Other promises helped me through the second series of radiation, even though it was a time of intense, overwhelming weakness and vomiting. I listened to Scriptures on healing—I read them over and over, and I prayed them out loud. But there was something in my heart I did not comprehend. Was I really expecting healing?

After hearing a lady's testimony about her disappointment in God when she wasn't healed, the Lord began uncovering an area of pain in my heart. Memories flooded my mind about my oldest daughter, Mary, who at the age of 6 developed juvenile diabetes. She was in the hospital over 50 days the first year. In those days, all testing had to be drawn from the vein; and I observed her writhe in pain over and over when they couldn't get the needle inserted into her tiny veins. I watched her suffer convulsions several times. Many emergency trips to the hospital resulted from the unavailability of good home testing equipment and the type of insulin used in the '60s and '70s.

At the time of the initial diagnosis, an older respected godly gentleman in our congregation fasted for several days and told us that the Lord was going to heal her. Even though we anticipated the healing, it never happened. Again, in her teens an immature believer told to her stop using insulin and trust God. She tried it, and everything went out of whack. I felt if there truly was healing, the doctors would be able to confirm it and take her off the medication.

I have witnessed many healings, some of them remarkable healings. At a meeting, I saw a man with a withered arm and hand instantly healed and come back to normal size. I prayed for a lady scheduled for surgery, and she was healed and did not have to go through surgery. Obviously it wasn't me; Jesus allowed me to be His vessel. Even though witnessing all these miracles, I could not understand why my daughter was not healed. Even a prominent prophet spoke over her that she would be healed before her second child was born, and it did not happen. We had prayed, fasted, anointed, confessed, trusted, cast out, and taken her numerous times to others for prayer. Through all this, a belief had taken hold in me that I didn't even realize. Simply described it was how could I expect healing for myself, after watching my little one suffer and not be healed?

In the midst of all my afflictions, I did not want to become offended in the Lord, for I was well aware of Jesus' reply to John the Baptist' messengers. Jesus was performing great miracles when the messengers asked Him if He was truly the one John prophesied was coming. Jesus told them to return to John and tell him how the blind see, the lame walk, the lepers are cleansed, and the deaf hear (Luke 7:22). But Jesus did not offer John a way out of his circumstances and stated, "*And blessed— happy [with life-joy and satisfaction in God's favor and salvation apart from outward conditions] and to be envied—-is he who takes no offense in Me and who is not hurt or resentful or annoyed or repelled or made to stumble, [whatever may occur]*" (Luke 7:23, Amplified). John was told about the wonderful miracles Jesus was doing, but he himself was not going to be gloriously delivered.

Maybe I did not expect glorious healing and deliverance from my situation; I do not know. However, there is a great deal of difference between what we call the faith of man in God and the faith of God imparted to man. It was far more important that I seek the Healer rather than healing and spend much time filling myself with His Word. All these were preparing me for the final release of a false premise. Each step has been important as well as praying in the Spirit as instructed by the psychologist. That prayer was beyond my understanding, and the Spirit was making intercession according to the will of the Father. The prayer went beyond my reasoning and pain. The answers and miracles that followed were not instantaneous but began and continued over a period of time. I am happy to report several miracles have taken place in my life within the last few months, and the pain is gone regarding my daughter's not being healed. Of course, I want to see her healed and continue to pray for her healing.

Pruning is God's way of cleaning out self-righteous thoughts such as personal views of how to function in His kingdom, personal motivations, personal pride, personal heritage, personal rights laid down for His rights and other's rights, personal offenses purged, complaints about leadership radically cut out, and any other area He chooses to clean out. From prison Paul wrote, "*I count all things loss for the excellence of the knowledge of Christ Jesus my Lord, for whom I have suffered the loss of all things, and count them as rubbish, that I may gain Christ*" (Philippians 3:8).

During pruning one may complain, compromise, rebel and demand one's own way, or run away. However, if we submit to the pruning, we will experience joy, comfort, and peace as we keep our eyes on Him, not on the pain. Pruning is not to prepare one to do more for Him, but to be in His presence more, to remain and abide in Him more. As Jesus continued his discourse with the disciples about the true vine and branches He emphasized the great importance of abiding in Him, for without

Him they could do nothing. (John 15:5) Their prayer life, their fruit bearing, and their love and joy were all connected to their abiding in Him.

Even though Satan is the destroyer, the Lord sovereignly uses our trials to draw us into a deeper relationship with Him. This pruning process is preparing the body of Christ for His return! In 1995, the Lord spoke to my heart from Daniel, that there would come a day when the compassion of the Lord will purify the hearts of men to the degree that great restoration will occur: "*And some of those of understanding shall fall, to refine them, purge them, and make them white, until the time of the end; because it is still for the appointed time*"(Daniel 11:38). Pruning or testing may continue for months or years. Joseph was tested for 13 years. After David's anointing to become king, he suffered many years of testing, and in the midst of it, he learned to "*strengthen himself in the Lord*" (I Samuel 30:6). When we submit to pruning, restoration will follow: restoration of yourself and the capacity to walk in love and forgiveness and restoration of others. In His final prayer before his betrayal and arrest, Jesus prayed, "*I am praying not only for these disciples but also for all who will ever believe in me, because of their testimony. My prayer for all of them is that they will be one, just as you and I are one, Father—-that just as you are in me and I am in you, so they will be in us, and the world will believe you sent me*" (John 17:20-21, NLT).

"Oh Father, may Jesus' prayer be fulfilled speedily! Fill us with your compassionate heart and cry for your body to become one in order that the world will be convinced you are the Messiah! Even so, come quickly, Lord Jesus!"

Building the Immune System

Chapter 14

In May, following my vascular surgery in January, I finally felt strong enough to make the trip to the Cancer Treatment Center in Tulsa for a checkup. At the last appointment in January, the medical oncologist had recommended six months of chemotherapy. In view of the fact that surgery immediately followed that appointment, I was unable to start that series of chemo. I wondered aloud to family and close friends if this was still on the agenda. My children and friends all strongly expressed their view that I should not submit to chemo at this time. In my heart I had determined to answer "not now" if I was pressed to undergo chemotherapy for six months. I was secure in God's love and confident in His peace, and *"Greater is He who is in me than he who is in the world"* (I John 4:4) regardless of circumstances. An excitement was birthed in my inner being and an assurance that I was going to receive a good report. What victory!

I had appointments with three doctors, and they were all amazed at the results of the tests that were taken and even more flabbergasted that I had lived through the surgery in January. The medical oncologist kept saying "God bless you," "God bless you," as he patted me. He went down through the pages of blood work and continued to say, "This is amazing!" Both he and his assistant commented on how wonderful it was to see good news, as they have to share so much bad news.

One doctor came to the waiting room in person with his arms outstretched to give me a big bear hug. He too was quite amazed at the blood work, as that is his specialty, and he recommended specific nutritional support to build the immune system. The Lord had not only brought me through a horrendous surgery, but He had also healed my body! No cancer could be found. Nurses, doctors, and staff took much pleasure and delight in this great miracle as well as I.

One doctor challenged me to prayerfully find answers from the Word and do research to strengthen my immune system. Cancer cells enter our body every day according to researchers. Paul has given us a divine order for dealing with life, "*may your whole spirit, soul, and body be preserved blameless at the coming of our Lord Jesus Christ*" (I Thessalonians 5:23b). The purpose of spirituality is to bring us into the image of Christ, not just to relieve us of some disease or stress in our life. I want to follow this prioritization of order in prayer, in thought, in life style, and in food. An entire chapter or book could easily be written on each area of the spirit, soul, and body; however, here are a few suggestions:

I. Spirit

Just because I have God's Word inside of me doesn't mean it's going to do the work. I must apply it to every situation. "*But be doers of the word, and not hearers only, deceiving yourselves*" (James 1:22). I am determined to know the Word and speak it, as it is greater than all my circumstances. As we yield to Him in increasing degrees of surrender and as we abide in Him and He abides in us, He brings forth His life in us. God's eternal purpose is to make man in His own image through Jesus Christ living within.

Moses expresses the Lord's heart towards His people when they are obedient to Him and keep all His commandments, all will go well with them and their children. This is reiterated several times in the book of Deuteronomy 5:29, 8:20; 11:13-28; 12:28; 15:6; 20:3-4; 28:13; 28:45-46, 58-59; plus this instruction, "*the word is very near you, in your mouth, and in your heart, that you may do it.... I have set before you life and death, blessing and cursing; therefore choose life, that both you and your descendants may* live." (Deuteronomy 30:14-19) Life is a choice! Every circumstance or situation presents us with that challenge: choose life or choose death. The following verses show various kinds of choices we need to make in order to remain healthy.

> "*A happy heart is good medicine and a cheerful mind works healing.*" (Proverbs 17:22a, Amplified)
> "*The joy of the Lord is your strength.*" (Nehemiah 8:10c)
> "*In Your presence is fullness of joy.*" (Psalm 15:11)
> "*A cheerful mind works healing.*" (Proverbs 17:22, Amplified)
> "*The fear of the Lord prolongs days.*" (Proverbs 10:27)
> "*He who waters will also be watered himself.*" (Proverbs 11:25) As one refreshes others, so he will be refreshed. See II Corinthians 9:6-11 for further explanation.
> "*Those who wait on the Lord shall renew their strength; they shall mount up with wings like eagles, they shall run and not be weary, they shall walk and not faint*" (Isaiah 40:31).
> "*...Drink deeply and be delighted with the abundance of his glory*" (Isaiah 66:10c).

Scriptures have been quoted in previous chapters and many more could be quoted regarding healing and health, but each individual needs to search the word for his/her own help. The attitude of the heart, the trust in the Lord, and the fresh revelation He inspires in our hearts from His Word continually builds our confidence in Him.

II. Soul

The mind, will, and emotions make up the soulish area. The soul has a tendency to react to the circumstances we are in. The devil tries to steal our hope; and when it seems to be fading away, we must "*bring every thought into captivity to the obedience of Christ*" (II Corinthians 10:5). The weapons of our warfare are not fleshly or physical "*but mighty in God for the destruction of strongholds*" (II Corinthians 10:4, Amplified). It is the Presence of the Lord Jesus that makes the weapons of our warfare mighty, empowering our words with authority as we pull down strongholds. Our minds must be transformed and completely renewed with new ideals and new attitudes, which include rejoicing. "*For in the time of trouble He shall hide me in His pavilion; in the secret place of His tabernacle He shall hide me; He shall set me high upon a rock. And now my head shall be lifted up above my enemies all around me; therefore I will offer sacrifices of joy in His tabernacle; I will sing, yes, I will sing praises to the Lord*" (Psalm 27:5-6). Rejoicing is a choice! As our will chooses to give a sacrifice of joy, the subsequent effect is a change in the mind and emotions.

King David practiced the art of encouraging himself by speaking to his soul, "*Why am I discouraged? Why so sad? I will put my hope in God! I will praise Him again—my Savior and my God*" (Psalms 42:5, 11, NLT)! In previous chapters we have discussed the importance of the tongue speaking words of life. Joel writes a proclamation and part of it states, "*Let the weak say, 'I am strong'*" (Joel 3:10). This has been a favorite quote of mine when asked how I was feeling, because it was obvious I was very weak. Now, I am saying, "I am stronger, praise the Lord!"

The Word indicates that laughter is good medicine. Laughter releases the stresses of the mind and restores our perspective. Even universities are teaching courses on the power of laughter. Norman Cousins wrote a book about the power of laughter after he was debilitated with a painful disease. He learned from experience that if he watched funny videos at least two hours, afterwards he could fall asleep without morphine.

For instance: A new pastor moved into town and went out one Saturday to visit his parishioners. All went well until he came to one house. It was obvious that someone was home, but no one came to the door even after he had knocked several times. Finally, he took out his card, wrote on the back, "Revelation 3:20" and stuck it in the door. The next day, as he was counting the offering, he found his card in the collection plate. Below his message was the notation, "Genesis 3:10." Revelation 3:20 reads: "Behold, I stand at the door and knock. If any man hear my voice, and opens, the door, I will come in to him, and will dine with him, and he with me." Genesis 3:10 read, "And he said, I heard thy voice in the garden, and I was afraid, because I was naked." I need to laugh heartily. I've learned that no matter how serious life is, I need a goofy friend. Find people that you can laugh with as part of building a vibrant support system.

At the Cancer Treatment Centers of America each patient is given a packet. In the handbook is a poem about cancer. It is thought provoking in that it challenges each one in their thought processes. Here it is:

What Cancer Cannot Do
Cancer is so limited
It cannot cripple love, it cannot
Shatter hope.
It cannot corrode faith, it cannot
Destroy peace.
It cannot kill friendship, it cannot
Suppress memories.
It cannot silence courage, it cannot
Invade the soul.

It cannot steal eternal life,
It cannot
Conquer the spirit.
Author Unknown

III. Body

I am not an expert in the area of nutritional support and supplements. I sought out a health practitioner, who is trained to evaluate the blood levels of nutrients, the body's ability to assimilate them (radiation has greatly affected assimilation in my body), and to indicate which nutrients I am deficient in. Also a trained nutritionist worked with my food program. I am trying to follow their recommendations for specific antioxidants and nutritional support. The immune system locates and destroys abnormal cells. Antioxidants in our body are countering the destructive forces of free radicals. Cancer cells siphon off nutrients for their own use, leaving the body in a weakened state, and radiation or chemotherapy also ravish the body, particularly the immune system.

The foundation of an anticancer diet is simple—vegetables and fruits. Plants contain copious amounts of cancer-fighting antioxidants and phytonutrients, compounds that protect plants from environmental damage. Researchers suggest that everyone eat at least five daily servings of vegetables and fruits and if possible eat organic food that is free from pesticides. Nutritionist recommend the following:

a. Cruciferous vegetables—broccoli, cabbage, cauliflower, Brussels sprouts, etc.
Colorful vegetables—dark leafy greens, orange—such as squash and sweet potatoes, and tomatoes.
b. Fruits—blueberries and raspberries are great cancer fighters. Citrus fruits have lots of vitamin C

    c.   High fiber—grains, skins of fruit and vegetables, fruit pectin and beans. The body needs at least 30 grams of fiber per day. The best sources of fiber are vegetables (especially beans), whole grains, fruits, and flaxseed.

    d.   Soy has powerful anticancer activity. Target isoflavone content—at least 50 mg per day. This can be gotten from ¼ cup textured soy protein, 1½ cup soy milk, ¾ cup tofu or tempeh, ½ cup cooked dried soy beans, or 3½ TB soy protein powder.

    e.   Keep intake of fat low—around 20 percent of total calories. Use olive oil for cooking. The best sources of omeg-3 fatty acids are cold-water fish and flaxseed.

    f.   Meat—buy organic whenever possible to avoid the excessive use of growth hormones and antibiotics given to animals in feed lots.

    g.   Water—drink 8 to 12 glasses daily. The body is mostly made up of water, and water is needed to flush out the toxins in the body.

Exercise at least 30 minutes three times a week. Start slowly and build up. I am trying to walk several days a week and increase the length of time as my strength improves.

It is important to remember that treatment and food choices are very personal. No one should pressure you to undertake a specific therapy. The only pressure you should feel is to educate yourself to the available options. The final choice lies with the patient, and it's a profoundly personal decision as there are many options for cancer treatments and no guarantees. The best choice, of course, is to work to avoid cancer altogether.

The way to realize God's ultimate victory is to reach toward His ultimate goal, which is complete transformation into the likeness of Christ. *"Beloved, I pray that you may prosper in all things and be in health, just as your soul prospers"* (III John 2).

God's Medicine

Chapter 15

A group of teenagers including my granddaughter were studying the book of James last summer. No one in the group personally knew anyone who had received a miraculous healing, and she wanted to know my thoughts on James 5:13-16 for their study. As I began to ponder that scripture and her questions, immediately the Spirit prompted me to read further.

Is anyone among you suffering? Let him pray. Is anyone cheerful? Let him sing psalms. Is anyone among you sick? Let him call for the elders of the church, and let them pray over him anointing him with oil in the name of the Lord. And the prayer of faith will save the sick, and the Lord will raise him up. And if he has committed sins, he will be forgiven. Confess your trespasses to one another, and pray for one another, that you may be healed. The effective, fervent prayer of a righteous man avails much. Elijah was a man with a nature like ours, and he prayed earnestly that it would not rain;

> ***and it did not rain on the land for three years and six months. And he prayed again, and the heaven gave rain, and the earth produced its fruit."***
> *(*James 5:13-18 NKJ*)*

Clearly Scriptures state that we need to confess our sins to each other and pray for each other so that we may be healed. But James reminds us to pray or travail fervently, and he uses the illustration of Elijah. What was there about Elijah's praying that might be important to healing? Let's go back to I Kings 18 and look at the situation. In the first verse of that chapter God gives direction to Elijah, "*Go, present yourself to Ahab, and I will send rain on the earth*" (I Kings 18:1 NKJ). The chapter describes the two bull offerings, one by the prophets of Baal and the other by Elijah. The prophets of Baal cried out all day to their false gods for fire to come down. They even cut themselves until the blood gushed out, but they received no answer. Then Elijah prepared his offering and asked them to fill their water pots and pour it on the wood three times. He called out to the Lord; and the fire of the Lord consumed the sacrifice, the wood, the stones, and licked up the water. Elijah tells Ahab to go home because rain is coming. But no rain is in sight. Elijah begins to pray. Why did he need to pray? The Lord already told him He was sending rain. He knew it was God's will for rain to come. He heard God speak it. How did he pray? What kind of praying did he do?

I love to ask the Lord questions. It seems to me that He delights in unfolding His ways and methods by revelation through His Word and the Holy Spirit to those who seek (and continue to seek).

Elijah knew it was God's will to break the 3½ years of drought. He understood God works through people. He took the posture of a woman giving birth of that era. He was in a "birthing" prayer on the mountain and he prayed seven times.

Seven is the number for completion in the Bible. Even though there was no sign of rain,

> *"Elijah went up to the top of Carmel; then he bowed down on the ground, and put his face between his knees, and said to his servant, "Go up now, look toward the sea." So he went up and looked, and said, "There is nothing." And seven times he went up and looked, and said, "There is nothing." And seven times he said, "Go again." Then it came to pass the seventh time, that he said, "There is a cloud, as small as a man's hand, rising out of the sea!" …. Now it happened in the meantime that the sky became black with clouds and wind, and there was heavy rain."*
> **(I Kings 18:42-45)**

James describes it as an effectual fervent or travailing prayer. It was a "birthing" prayer by the spirit. Paul also gives us the picture of birthing prayer in his writings, *"My little children, for whom I labor in birth again until Christ is formed in you"* (Galations 4:19).

Another Biblical example, which supports the premise for the need of prayer when God's will is already known, is found in Daniel chapter 9. While Daniel was studying the writings of the prophet Jeremiah, he learned that Jerusalem and Israel would be under siege for 70 years. Daniel realized the duration of the captivity was complete. What he did with that promise is a key for us when we know God's will or receive a promise. He did not sit idly waiting for Israel's deliverance. Immediately Daniel began to fast and pray. He even wore rough sackcloth and sprinkled himself with ashes. Apparently, he knew that God wanted his involvement.

His prayer covered four areas:

1. He exalted the awesomeness and greatness of God and proclaimed His unfailing love and mercy.
2. He confessed Israel's sin and rebellion.
3. He acknowledges the Lord's righteousness and pleads for mercy.
4. He asks the Lord to hear, forgive, listen, and act for His name's sake.

> *"O Lord, hear! O Lord, forgive! O Lord, listen and act! Do not delay for Your own sake, my God, for Your city and Your people are called by Your name."*
>
> ## (Daniel 9:19)

After Daniel's prayer, the angel Gabriel came to give him insight and understanding. God had made the decision in heaven and prophesied it through Jeremiah. But a man was needed to "birth," "travail," or "enforce" that decision on earth by prayer and faith by the Spirit.

Elijah and Daniel as human beings could not produce results, but their prayers released the Holy Spirit to do a work. The Lord wants our active involvement in birthing His will. James sufficiently gives direction to one type of healing. It is God's will to heal by calling the "*elders of the ecclesia, and let them pray over him rubbing him with olive oil in the name of the Lord.*" (James 5:14, Concordant Literal New Testament) May we be inspired and challenged by the "keys" in prayers offered by

Daniel and Elijah. This is by no means an exhaustive study of birthing prayer, but hopefully, it is enough to begin new revelation in our prayer life. I'm completely convinced healing in my body came through the fervent birthing prayers of God's people. They knew it was God's will to heal, and they didn't let go.

I have an unshakable confidence in the Word of God, and I continue to read or quote many healing scriptures to build and preserve my faith. Three areas are crucial in my walk with the Lord:

1) **Plead the blood of Jesus over myself**
2) **Pray in the spirit daily**
3) **Read, believe, speak, and apply the Word daily**

Scriptures that I quote or refer to frequently are listed below. May I suggest you record these onto a tape or purchase tapes of healing scriptures. As you listen to them, you will soon be able to quote the verses, and they will become part of your thought life as well as minister life to you.

1. **Give attention and listen carefully to God's Word. It will be life to you.**

> My son, pay attention to what I say; listen closely to my words,
> Do not let them out of your sight, keep them within your heart,
> For they are life to those who find them and [radiant] health to a man's whole body.
> Proverbs 4:20-22, NIV (radiant from the Living Bible)

> He said, "If you listen carefully to the voice of the Lord your God and do what is right in his eyes, if your pay attention to his commands and

79

keep all his decrees, I will not bring on you any of the diseases I brought on the Egyptians, for I am the Lord who heals you."
Exodus 15:26, NIV

Blessed is the man who listens to me, watching daily at my doors, waiting at my doorway. For whoever find me finds life [health] and receives favor from the Lord.
Proverbs 8:35, NIV

2. Worship and praise the Lord and He will keep you.

Worship the Lord your God, and his blessing will be on your food and water. I will take away sickness from among you.
Exodus 23:25, NIV

The Lord will keep you free from every disease. He will not inflict on you the horrible disease you knew in Egypt, but He will inflict them on all who hate him.
Deuteronomy 7:15, NIV

Praise the Lord, O my soul; all my inmost being, praise his holy name.
Praise the Lord, O my soul, and forget not all his benefits.
He forgives all my sins and heals all my diseases. He redeems my life from the pit and crowns me with love and compassion. He satisfies my desires with good things, so that my youth is renewed like the eagles.
Psalm 103:1-5, NIV

3. **Jesus paid the price for our healing for by His stripes we are healed**.

> Surely He took up our infirmities and carried our sorrows, yet we considered him stricken by God, smitten by Him, and afflicted.
> But He was pierced for our transgressions, He was crushed for our iniquities; the punishment that brought us peace was upon Him and by His wounds we are healed.
> Isaiah 53:4-5, NIV

> Who Himself bore our sins in His own body on the tree, that we, having died to sins, might live for righteousness—-by whose stripes you were healed.
> I Peter 2:24, NKJ

4. **What you say and think is vitally important! It produces life or death!**

> The tongue of the wise brings healing.
> Proverbs 12:18, NIV

> A wholesome tongue is a tree of life
> Proverbs 15:4, NKJ

> A happy heart is a good medicine and a cheerful mind works healing.
> Proverbs 17:22, Amplified

> The tongue has the power of life and death, and those who love it will eat its fruit.
> Proverbs 18:21, NIV

5. Reverence and respect the Lord for it leads to life.

The fear of the Lord leads to life [health].
Proverbs 19:23, NIV

Humility and the fear of the Lord bring wealth and honor and life [health].
Proverbs 22:4, NIV

Trust in the Lord, and do good; dwell in the land, and feed on His faithfulness. Delight yourself also in the Lord, and He shall give you the desires of your heart. Commit your way to the Lord, trust also in Him.
Psalm 37:3-5, NKJ

For the Lord God is a sun and shield; the Lord will give grace and glory; no good thing will He withhold from those who walk uprightly.
Psalm 84:11, NKJ

The labor of the righteous leads to life [health].
The fear of the Lord prolongs days.
The way of the Lord is strength for the upright.
Proverbs 10:16, 27, 29, NIV

6. His Word produces life!

He sent forth His word and healed them; He rescued them from the grave.
Psalm 107:20, NIV

He taught me and said, "Lay hold of my words with all your heart; keep my commands and you will live."
Proverbs 4:4, NIV

Revive me according to Your Word.
Psalm 119:25, 107, 149, 154, NKJ

This is my comfort in my affliction, for Your Word has given me life.
Psalm 119:50, NKJ

If your law had not been my delight, I would have perished in my affliction.
Psalm 119:92, NKJ

Many are the afflictions of the righteous, but the Lord delivers him out of them all.
Psalm 34:19, NKJ

He heals the brokenhearted and binds up their wounds.
Psalm 147:3, NIV

7. Give Him all your anxious worries! He is your source!

God is our refuge and strength, an ever-present help in trouble.
Psalm 46:1, NIV

Cast your cares on the Lord and He will sustain you; He will never let the righteous fall.
Psalm 55:22, NIV

Cast all your anxiety on him because he cares for you.

I Peter 5:7, NIV

Jabez was more honorable than his brothers…he cried out to the God of Israel, 'Oh that you would bless me and enlarge my territory! Let your hand be with me, and keep me from harm so that I will be free from pain.' And God granted his request.

I Chronicles 4:9—10, NIV

8. Jesus healed the sick!

That evening after sunset the people brought to Jesus all the sick and demon-possessed. The whole town gathered at the door, and Jesus healed many who had various diseases. He also drove out many demons, but he would not let the demons speak because they knew who he was.

Mark 1:32-34, NIV

Jesus sent the disciples out two by two. "So they went out and preached that people should repent. And they cast out many demons, and anointed with oil many who were sick, and healed them."

Mark 6:12-13, NKJ (also see Matthew 10)

And He cast out the spirits with a word, and healed all who were sick.

Matthew 8:16, NKJ

Then great multitudes came to Him, having with them those who were lame, blind, mute, maimed, and many others; and they laid them down at Jesus' feet, and He healed them. So the multitude marveled when they saw the mute speaking, the maimed made whole, the lame walking, and the blind seeing; and they glorified the God of Israel.

Matthew 15:30-31, NKJ

9. Through the apostles many were healed!

And through the hands of the apostles many signs and wonders were done among the people. Also a multitude gathered from the surrounding cities to Jerusalem, bringing sick people and those who were tormented by unclean spirits, and they were all healed.

Acts 5:12, 16, NKJ

Now God worked unusual miracles by the hands of Paul, so that even handkerchiefs or aprons were brought from his body to the sick, and the disease left them and the evil spirits went out of them.

Acts 19:11-12, NKJ

Paul went in to him and prayed, and he laid his hands on him and healed him. So when this was done, the rest of those on the island who had diseases also came and were healed.

Acts 28:8-9, NKJ

10. The elders in the local church anoint with oil and the sick are made whole.

Is any of you sick? He should call the elders of the church to pray over him and anoint him with oil in the name of the Lord. And the prayer offered in faith will make the sick person well; the Lord will raise him up.

James 5:14-15, NIV

11. Confession: Jesus Christ never changes!

For with God nothing will be impossible.

Luke 1:37, NIV

I shall not die, but live and declare the works of the Lord.

Psalm 118:17, NKJ

Jesus Christ is the same yesterday, today, and forever.

Hebrews 13:8, NKJ

I tell you the truth, anyone who has faith in me will do what I have been doing. He will do even greater things than these, because I am going to the Father. And I will do whatever you ask in My name, so that the Son may bring glory to the Father. You may ask me for anything in My name, and I will do it.

John 14:12-15, NIV

He who is in you is greater than he who is in the world.

I John 4:4, NKJ

And if the Spirit of Him who raised Jesus from the dead is living in you, He who raised Christ from the dead will also give life to your mortal bodies through His Spirit who lives in you.

Romans 8:11, NIV

How great is our Lord! His power is absolute! His understanding is beyond comprehension!
Psalm 147:5, NLT

Affliction will not rise up a second time.
Nahum 1:9, NKJ

I would have lost heart, unless I had believed that I would see the goodness of the Lord in the land of the living. Wait on the Lord and be of good courage. And He shall strengthen your heat; wait, I say, on the Lord!
Psalm 27:13-14, NKJ

Ruth E. Foat

Epilogue

"So be truly glad! There is wonderful joy ahead, even though it is necessary for you to endure many trials for a while. These trials are only to test your faith, to show that it is strong and pure. It is being tested as fire tests and purifies gold—and your faith is far more precious to God than mere gold. So if your faith remains strong after being tried by fiery trials, it will bring you much praise and glory and honor on the day when Jesus Christ is revealed to the whole world."
(I Peter 1:6-7 NLT)

Change may come through prayer or it may come through praise. Sometimes change takes place under godly counselors such as I experienced at the Cancer Center. Changed attitudes may develop while truly seeking forgiveness or while forgiving others. Impurities are cleansed in the midst of fiery trials as one submits to Jesus Christ. These changes did not make me "holier" than anyone else, but it changed me and taught me many things. I am still learning. I am still changing. Paul best describes my feelings,

> *"I don't mean to say that I have already achieved these things or that I have already reached perfection! But I keep working toward that day when I will finally be all that Christ Jesus saved me for and wants me to be. No, dear brothers and sisters, I am still not all I should be, but I am focusing all my energies on this one thing: Forgetting the past and looking forward to what lies ahead, I strain to reach the end of the race and receive the prize for which God, through Christ Jesus, is calling us up to heaven."* **(Philippians 3:12-14 NLT)**

I have tried to be transparent, open, and willing to allow others to peer into my life and see my imperfections, trials, corrections, and victories. I do not regret opening myself to the searching work of God. Yes, it is painful, but the peace and freedom is worth it.

I used to spend the fall season dreading the coming winter and wondering how cold and nasty it might be. The ten weeks at the Cancer Treatment Center totally wiped out fall last year. But what a change this year! When I stepped outdoors in September an exuberant joy rushed through me! The sky looked bluer, the grass looked greener, and the geraniums looked bigger and redder. Fall is wonderful!

Family has become more precious. Friends are more valuable and dear. Strife seems so utterly useless. Differing viewpoints don't matter. Stuff has lost its importance. I pray that the Kingdom of God will come soon and that His will be done here on earth, just as it is in heaven. I want to know Christ more and experience the mighty power that raised him from the dead. I have openly shared with you in the hope that my experiences will strengthen you.

Ruth E. Foat

About the Author

Ruth was raised on a farm in Iowa, learning to milk cows, feed pigs, drive the tractor, tend a garden, cook, sew, and play the piano—a great old-fashioned work ethic. Sunday afternoons were the highlight of the week, with games played together or sitting around Mother listening to her read. Her parents encouraged her to memorize 500 Scripture verses to win a trip to camp.

She attended Vennard College in University Park, Iowa, and completed her studies for ordination. Along with her husband, they pastored churches in North Dakota, Iowa, Oregon, and Minnesota. She has been a speaker for Women's Aglow groups in several states, Marriage Enrichment Seminars, and Mother's Day banquets plus leading Bible Studies in her local church and area. In Atlanta, she was the Registrar for a Bible College. Ruth Foat was a minister for thirty years before the physical attacks on her body.

She has lived what she writes. And, she says she is still learning. She is the mother of four children and eight grandchildren. She and her husband live in Mason City, Iowa.